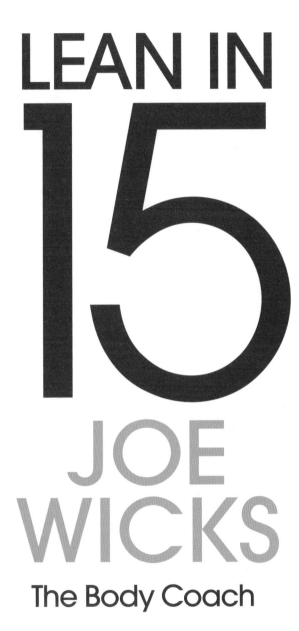

LEAN IN 15

JOE WICKS

The Body Coach

WILLIAM MORROW

An Imprint of HarperCollins*Publishers*

This book is written as a source of information only. The information contained in this book should by no means be considered a substitute for the advice of your qualified medical professional, who should always be consulted before beginning any new diet, exercise or other health program.

HarperCollins books may be purchased for educational, business, or sales promotional use. For information please e-mail the Special Markets Department at SPsales@harpercollins.com.

Originally published in the United Kingdom in 2015 by Bluebird, an imprint of Pan Macmillan.

FIRST U.S. EDITION

Designed and Typeset by www.cabinlondon.co.uk
Food photography and images on pages 4, 29, 115, 184 © Maja Smend
Fitness photography in Chapter 6 and images on pages 10–11, 22–3, 30–1, 100–01, 166–7, 192–3, 204–5, 212, 221 © Glen Burrows

Grateful acknowledgment is made to "My Lean Winners" and the "Lean in 15 Heroes" for permission to include the images on pages 207–11 and 216–17.

Library of Congress Cataloging-in-Publication Data has been applied for.

ISBN 978-0-06-249366-8

16 17 18 19 20 OV/QGT 10 9 8 7 6 5 4 3 2

CONTENTS

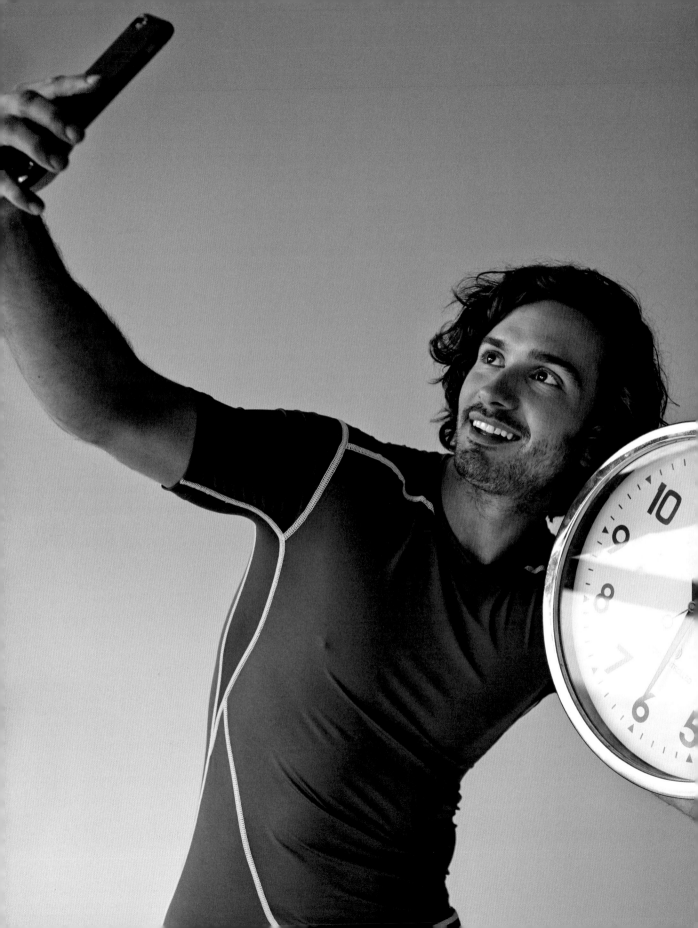

A LITTLE BIT ABOUT ME

//

When I posted my first ever #Leanin15 video on Instagram in early 2014, I never imagined it would lead to me writing this book. It all started as a bit of fun in my kitchen, with the idea of sharing simple recipes to help people get lean.

All of the meals were ready in 15 minutes, and the videos were only 15 seconds long . . . hence the hashtag #Leanin15. To begin with, no one was watching my videos, and my neighbors thought I was mad. They often heard me singing or shouting, "Bosh, that's Lean in 15" and "Oooh, midget trees" (that's what I call broccoli, by the way!).

Some of my friends thought it was stupid, and said I should get back to doing personal training and running my boot camps—that's what I had been happily doing for the past 5 years. But I was having fun, so I just carried on anyway, often posting up to 3 videos a day. It took a lot of time and energy to stop and film everything I cooked, but I saw every meal as an opportunity to share a new recipe, and this was my motivation to keep going.

> " I saw every meal as an opportunity to share a new recipe "

To my surprise, within a few months, hundreds of thousands of people all over the world were following along, making my recipes at home and sharing them online. I think the speed and simplicity of my meals, along with the fact that I was clearly enjoying myself, inspired so many people to get involved.

I'm completely self-taught when it comes to cooking, so I never overcomplicate things. I use foods that anyone can find in their local supermarket and this makes Lean in 15 accessible to everyone and perfect for busy people.

My approach is also about making small lifestyle changes rather than following a strict regime. I often post photos of myself eating out in restaurants and enjoying treats. I do love a chocolate lava cake—guilty as charged!

I think people respond well to me because I don't eat perfectly all the time and I never pretend that I do. In fact, my diet used to be pretty shocking. I've always trained hard, but I didn't really take my nutrition seriously. Like most busy people, I was lazy when it came to cooking and used lack of time as an excuse. I often ate cereal, sandwiches on the go and prepared meals. This left me feeling tired, but I just accepted it as normal. I drank fizzy drinks and snacked on chocolate bars in between personal training clients. During this time, my body didn't change much and I could never get lean. Eventually, I discovered that no matter how hard I trained, I couldn't out-train a poor diet.

It was only when I really started to study nutrition after college that I realized just how important real food was for my energy levels and making changes in my body. The more I understood, the more I started to transform my own body. With this new knowledge and understanding of nutrition, I was able to get lean and stay lean. I then started to apply my knowledge with my clients, and it was remarkable how quickly their bodies would respond. Helping clients get fast transformations meant I soon got fully booked as a personal trainer. But, even with two busy

> **My approach is also about making small lifestyle changes rather than a strict regime**

boot camps, I could only ever work with about 100 people each week. This wasn't enough for me. I wanted to help more people reach their goals, so I started putting more energy into my social media. With Twitter, Facebook, YouTube and Instagram, I was able to reach thousands of people at once by sharing content online—video recipes, workouts and blogs. As my social media following grew, I started to realize just how shocking the diet industry really was. Every day I would receive messages from people on all sorts of depressing low-calorie crash diets, and it soon became apparent just how much wrong information people were being given—and how far they were willing to go to lose weight. Regimes of training for 2 hours a day and eating fewer than 1,000 calories were way too common, and it upset me that people were living this way, always trying to find a shortcut and never getting the results they wanted. Very unhappy people were being held prisoner by diets that would never give them the lean body they wanted. I believe such crash diets are a contributory factor to so many of the eating disorders and body image issues we face today. People have become convinced that the only way to lose body fat is to drastically cut calories to create a huge energy deficit—but this only leads to yo-yo dieting and people battling their weight for years, which is not a healthy way to live, and it shouldn't be accepted as the norm.

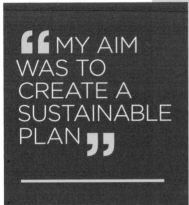

"MY AIM WAS TO CREATE A SUSTAINABLE PLAN"

One day while I was out jogging, I decided I would do something about it. I would create an online nutrition and training plan to educate people properly and rescue them from these damaging, unhealthy diets. My aim was to create a sustainable plan with tasty meals that would get people eating more food, training more effectively (and for much less time!) and burning fat.

Everyone has different energy demands. My meal plans are unique; I create tailored meal plans that allow choice and flexibility, to ensure people get results and keep them. After months of planning, the 90 Day Shift, Shape and Sustain plan was born. I used social media to promote it, and started to post "before" and "after" transformation pictures, along with written testimonials. I had no idea what I had created at the time—and, to this day, I can't quite believe the success it's had. But by creating an online community, I unknowingly connected thousands of people who were all on the same journey. As more and more clients signed up online, I had to step away from my boot camps, and eventually I passed on all my personal training clients to a friend. My business was now fully online and going global.

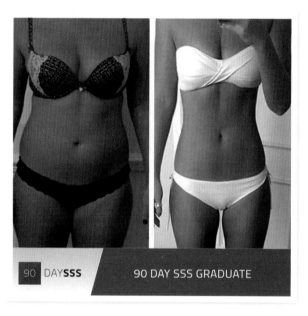

90 DAY**SSS**   90 DAY SSS GRADUATE

Originally it was mainly people from the UK signing up, but then people all over the world started to get on board. Places as far away as Australia, Sweden, Singapore and Dubai were starting to hear about Lean in 15 and signing up to my 90 Day Shift, Shape and Sustain plan. It started off with just me answering a few emails and sending a few plans out each week, but before I knew it I had thousands of people signing up each month and a team of support staff to help coach clients on their journey.

I absolutely love what I do now, and although I never get to actually meet any of my clients, I'm really proud of all of them and feel inspired by them every day. By educating people on nutrition I have been able to empower them to take control and achieve their goals in a healthy and enjoyable way.

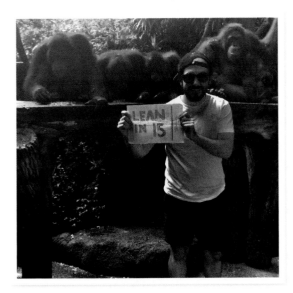

> **❝ I am now on a mission to help even more people ❞**

As The Body Coach, I am now on a mission to help even more people. It's important to note that my online business didn't just happen overnight—it grew organically and came from nothing but hard work. It takes a lot of trust for a person to buy into something without ever meeting you, and I built that trust up over hundreds of hours of interaction, videos and tweets. When no one was listening, I kept sharing and giving, and eventually people started to hear me.

So that's a little bit about me and my story up to now. I'm very excited to be sharing my knowledge and recipes with you. I hope you enjoy the book and get inspired to cook, prep like a boss and get the body you've always wanted.

Joe Wicks

—THE BODY COACH

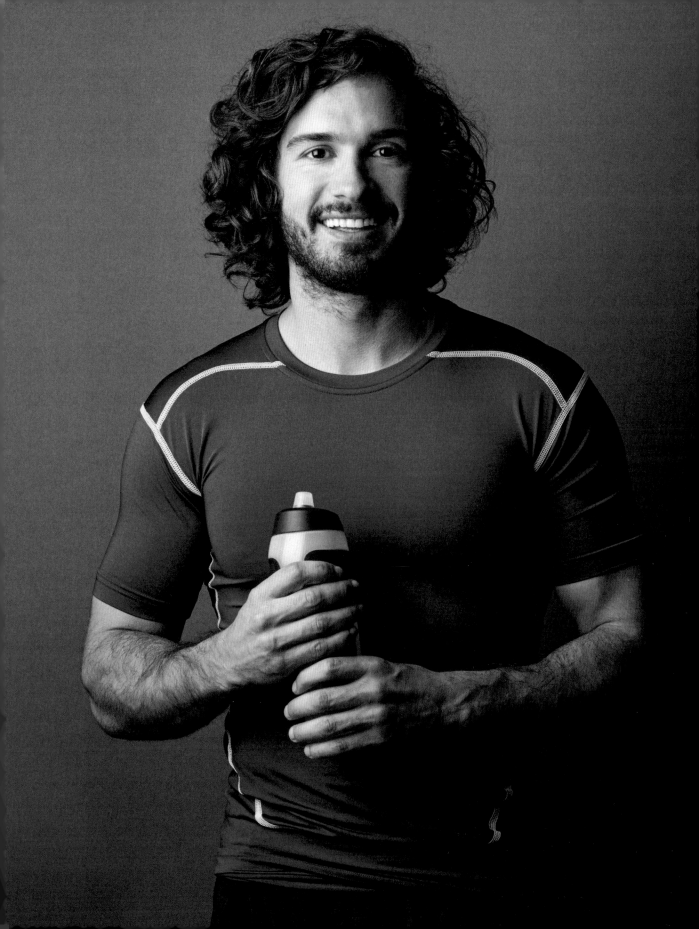

THE LEAN IN 15 PLAN

DIETS DON'T WORK!

///

The problem with diets is that they don't work—not in the long term, anyway. Yes, you can lose weight initially, especially with a drastic decrease in calories, but the likelihood is that you will soon return to your old eating habits and regain any weight lost. After working with thousands of clients, I know that success only happens when a program is enjoyable and sustainable. A meal plan needs to be easy to follow and stress-free, because life is stressful enough and we simply don't have the time to spend hours in the kitchen every day.

This is why I created Lean in 15. No matter how busy you are, you can take control and find a quarter of an hour to cook your meals and stay lean. This isn't a strict diet—it's a lifestyle that will transform your body and the way you eat forever. Once I teach you how to fuel your body properly, you will never need to follow a low-calorie diet again.

Most of the recipes in this book will be ready in less than 15 minutes, and many of them can be batch-cooked, so you can double up and prepare meals for the day or week ahead. A few of the meals take a little longer than 15 minutes so are not technically "Lean in 15" but don't worry, it's because they taste great and will be well worth the wait! The busier you are, the

> " Success only happens when a program is enjoyable and sustainable ""

more you will need to prep your meals. I call this "prepping like a boss," and it's one of the ways you can guarantee your success. I'll be sharing my top tips for prepping like a boss further on in this book, so keep a lookout.

There are no shortcuts

I want you to ignore all the ads trying to sell you fat-burning herbal supplements, meal-replacement shakes or juice diets. They are not the solution. In fact, these diets are the problem, as they go against the basic principles of nutrition and the way metabolism works. What's more, they rely on repeat business, because they know that once you lose the weight, you'll soon regain it and be back for more of their products. I want to help you break this vicious circle once and for all.

The truth is there are no shortcuts to a lean body. It takes time, dedication, consistent training and the right nutrition. The good news is that Lean in 15 is not going to deprive you of entire food groups or leave you feeling hungry like most diets. My approach is the complete opposite. I want to encourage you to think differently and change your approach. I want you to eat *more* food, and I'm going to show you how to fuel your body properly, so you burn fat and build lean muscle. The more lean muscle you have, the more efficient your metabolism will be—and that means you can enjoy eating even more food. That's winning!

I'm also going to explain the importance of fats, proteins and carbohydrates, so you understand what to fuel your body with and when. My philosophy is simple and easy to adopt into your lifestyle.

> **I want you to eat *more* food, and I'm going to show you how to fuel your body properly**

Your body is unique

The portions in the recipes in this book are not specifically tailored to you, as it would be impossible without knowing much more about you (your current weight, activity level, age range and more). Every body has its own unique energy demands, so you will need to increase or decrease the portion sizes according to your activity levels. For example, if you train hard and have a really physically active job, you need to eat more than someone who sits at a desk for eight hours a day and does little exercise.

It doesn't have to be difficult or complicated. You will soon start to notice if you feel energized or not, so listen to your body—and please don't go hungry! Although I can't tailor portion sizes to individual readers, the structured way of eating outlined in this book—what to eat and when—is very effective for fat loss. The structure is the same as cycle one of my 90 Day Shift, Shape and Sustain plan, which has worked brilliantly for tens of thousands of people. This phase is called the "Shift" phase, because that's exactly what it does. It shifts unwanted fat by putting your body in fat-burning mode at all times through a combination of diet and exercise (I have also included some sample home HIIT workouts for you to try out—see page 194).

Understanding macronutrients

Our three main energy sources—fats, protein and carbohydrates—are called macronutrients. They all play an important role in helping our bodies stay lean, strong and healthy. The way of eating in this book won't cut any of these out of your diet, but rather will provide you with them in the right ratios at the right time to get the best possible response from your body.

During low-intensity activity, such as watching TV, walking to stores and even sleeping, your body mostly uses fats to fuel itself. When working at a high intensity, it mostly uses stored carbohydrates for energy. I'm going to show you how to use this knowledge to your advantage, to ensure your body is always using the correct energy source in line with your energy demands.

Let's talk about fats

Fats have been unfairly demonized, to the extent that people now believe that all fats are bad and will make you get fat, and a whole industry has risen around low-fat versions of common foods. Fat is often the first thing people cut out when trying to lose weight. But not all fats are the same. Some fats—such as trans-fats found in processed foods—should be avoided, but others are actually essential for the body, such as omega-3s (found in oily fish), which help reduce inflammation. These are known as essential fatty acids (EFAs), as they cannot be made in the body and so must be obtained from the diet. Fat also plays

" Listen to your body—and please don't go hungry "

an essential role in vitamin absorption: vitamins A, D, E and K are fat-soluble, meaning your body can't absorb them without fat being present.

People also often associate energy with carbohydrates, but fats are actually the most energy-dense macronutrient of all. Fats provide your body with 9 calories energy per gram, compared to just 4 calories per gram from protein and carbohydrates. This makes fat an incredible energy source, and one that keeps blood sugar levels stable. Fat also takes longer to digest in the body, which means you feel satisfied for longer and are less likely to snack in between meals.

Why are fats important?

Fats have several important roles in the body, including:
- ★ Providing you with energy
- ★ Enabling the absorption of fat-soluble vitamins
- ★ Protecting your organs, nerves and tissues
- ★ Helping to regulate body temperature
- ★ Every cell membrane in the body needs fat for protection, and fat is also needed to grow new healthy cells
- ★ Fats are involved in the production of essential hormones in the body
- ★ Maintenance of healthy hair, skin and nails

What are the types of fat?

There are 3 types of fat:
- ★ Saturated—animal fats, butter, eggs, cheese, coconut oil
- ★ Monounsaturated—nuts, avocados, extra virgin olive oil, peanut oil, sesame oil
- ★ Polyunsaturated—sunflower oil, walnut oil, flaxseed oil, and oily fish such as salmon and mackerel

Saturated fats have an awful reputation, which dates back to the 1950s, when a study found that the consumption of saturated fat increased levels of bad cholesterol in the blood, and that this led to coronary heart disease. In hindsight, this research was extremely flawed and failed to take into account those countries where people had a very high intake of saturated fat and yet very low levels of heart disease. Unfortunately this "diet-heart" hypothesis influenced government health guidelines and the low-fat food industry started to boom. Instead of fats, we were encouraged to consume more carbohydrates, such as grains, rice and pasta. But since then, deaths from obesity, diabetes and heart disease have continued to rise.

Ironically, the latest research suggests that saturated fats from butter, milk, cream, eggs and coconut oil actually increase the levels of good cholesterol in the blood and benefit the heart, so there is no need to fear these foods. This doesn't mean you should sit down and eat a whole wheel of cheese, though. Fats do contain lots of calories, after all, so you need to eat everything in moderation and in line with your own personal energy demands.

Monounsaturated fats

Monounsaturated fats, found in things such as extra virgin olive oil, avocados and nuts, are great for increasing good cholesterol levels. This is one of the reasons a handful of nuts or seeds, or half an avocado makes a perfect snack. Unlike sugary cereal bars and chocolate, these snacks will also keep your blood sugar levels stable and sustain your energy levels for much longer.

Polyunsaturated fats

Polyunsaturated fats can be found in oily fish like salmon and mackerel and are a great source of omega-3 fatty acids. These are considered anti-inflammatory, which means they reduce your risk of injuries and chronic disease. I'm not the biggest fan of fish, and for the first 25 years of my life I wouldn't go near it, but I've slowly trained myself to eat it because I understand its importance for my health. No amount of omega-3 fish oil capsules will beat a fresh piece of wild salmon, so try to eat fish at least twice a week.

Bad fats

The hydrogenated fats we need to eliminate from our diet aren't just found in sugary sweets, pastries and fast-food restaurants. They are also hidden in many low-fat diet products. Low-fat prepared meals, for example, may be low in saturated fat

" **A handful of nuts or seeds, or half an avocado makes a perfect snack** " but they are often loaded with hydrogenated trans-fats to increase their shelf-life. My advice is to prepare all of your own meals from scratch, avoiding packaged meals wherever possible.

What should I cook with?

You'll notice that I mostly use coconut oil or butter for cooking— this is because these saturated fats are more stable when heated to high temperatures. Processed polyunsaturated vegetable oils and margarines, on the other hand, become unstable when heated. This means they oxidize easily, producing free radicals, and these are not what you want to be putting inside your body. When free radicals attack fat molecules, they develop similar properties to a trans-fat, increasing the levels of bad cholesterol in your blood at the same time as decreasing the levels of good cholesterol—a double-whammy effect that's not great when it comes to the health of your heart.

What about protein?

Protein forms the basis of all meals in the Lean in 15 plan, and remains consistent on both training and rest days. Protein is essential for:

★ Maintaining the structure and strength of cells and tissues
★ Regulation of metabolism
★ Production of hormones
★ Repair and growth of muscle tissues
★ Strengthening your immune system

Where should I get my protein?

Proteins are broken down into amino acids inside the body. Many of my recipes contain animal protein sources, such as eggs, fish, chicken and beef. These are considered complete protein sources because they contain all the essential amino acids needed by the body. If you are a vegetarian you can of course use tofu or other soy-based meat substitutes as a protein source, but you'll need to eat much larger quantities to get your protein intake to the required level.

> " Prepare all of your own meals from scratch, avoiding packaged meals wherever possible "

Protein powder

I always say real food, not dust, burns fat. What I mean by this is that supplements should only be used alongside a good diet and not in place of real food. However, you may notice that in some of my recipes, such as overnight oats, I do use protein powder. Whey protein is a brilliant post-workout addition to your diet because it reaches the muscles quickly, so the amino acids can start to repair and rebuild muscle fibers immediately after a training session. If you need a dairy-free alternative (whey is derived from dairy), you could try a vegan protein powder, such as hemp or pea.

Let's talk about carbohydrates

There is so much confusion surrounding carbohydrates—which carbs are good and which are bad, and when you can and can't eat them. I'm going to clear all this up and show you what a great energy source they can be.

We've all heard the ridiculous myth that eating carbs after 6 P.M. makes you fat. It's pure nonsense! Carbs don't make you fat. What actually makes us gain fat is when we eat over and above our bodies' energy demands. So, provided you eat the right amount each day, you will not gain fat but instead will be able to train harder and build more muscle, which will make you leaner.

Why do we need carbohydrates?

★ Carbohydrates are the main source of energy for muscles during intense exercise
★ They are needed for the proper functioning of the central nervous system, kidneys and muscles
★ Carbs also contain fiber, which is important for good intestinal health and digestion
★ They are essential for healthy brain function

The white carb police

Lots of people seem to be scared of eating white bread, pasta and rice, and attempt to ban them from their lives. I call these

> "REAL FOOD, NOT DUST, BURNS FAT"

people "the white carb police." Unshakeable in their belief that you can't eat white carbs when trying to burn fat, they will eat only the brown, whole-grain versions of these carbs—but you really don't need to fear white carbs.

While it's true that whole-grain carbs have a lower glycemic load (GL), which means they don't cause your blood sugar levels to spike as much as white carbs, after training your body actually loves high-GL foods. The higher the GL of a food, the greater will be the elevation of blood glucose levels, prompting the pancreas to release insulin. However, this insulin response is great after a workout as it means the nutrients from your carbohydrate-refuel meal are shuttled to the muscles quicker. Combining high-GL carbs with low-GL carbs such as table sugar with porridge oats reduces the overall GL and elevation of blood sugar levels.

In summary, if you love brown rice, eat brown rice—but if you long for a big bowl of white rice or a white bagel, then know that after you train is the ideal time to enjoy it.

How will I be eating?

. . . .

You are going to be eating in line with your energy demands. This means that you will eat differently on training days and rest days.

You are going to ensure that your body is using the correct energy source, in line with your energy demands—that is, carbohydrates after exercise, and fats as steady fuel for the remainder of your day and night, and on rest days.

The recipes in this book are broken down into 3 sections:
1. Reduced-carbohydrate meals: rich in healthy fats and protein
2. Post-workout carbohydrate-refuel meals: high in protein and carbohydrates
3. Snacks and treats: sweet and savory snacks and tasty treats

On a training day, you will eat 2 reduced-carbohydrate meals, 1 post-workout carbohydrate-refuel meal and 2 snacks.

On a rest day, you will eat 3 reduced-carbohydrate meals and 2 snacks.

> " You will eat differently on training days and rest days "

Why do I eat this way?

My post-workout carbohydrate-refuel meal structure is very effective for fat loss. Your body stores carbohydrates in the liver and muscles as glycogen and, after a workout, these are depleted, so you need to "refuel" and top up those stores after training. When you consume carbohydrates, they are broken down into sugars and this increases your blood sugar levels, causing the pancreas to release insulin. Remember, this is a good thing post-workout as insulin shuttles the nutrients from your meal into your muscles quickly, so they can get to work repairing and rebuilding.

Whenever you're not working intensively, your body uses mainly fats for fuel. This is why you will reduce your carbohydrates on rest days and increase your fat intake. At first you might struggle to make this change. Psychologically you may feel like you are low on energy, but don't forget you are still providing your body with energy—just from fats instead of carbs. You will soon adjust to it, so persevere. And remember, you are eating to stay lean.

What meals should I choose?

The training plan is flexible and all meals are interchangeable. This means you could have protein pancakes for breakfast or dinner, depending on when you train. Just remember that you are "earning" those carbs during your workout, so you must always choose a carbohydrate-refuel meal afterward, regardless of how late you train.

If there is a recipe you want to try, but you don't like a certain ingredient, such as onions or peppers, simply swap it for something similar that you do enjoy. The same goes with the protein—for example, if you don't like ground beef, you can always use ground turkey.

I've included a few treats in the book but these should only be eaten once or twice a week and only after a workout.

Alcohol and fat loss

. . . .

I'm always very honest and realistic with my clients when it comes to drinking alcohol. I never tell them to cut it out completely, as this is a personal choice for them to make. I just remind them that the less booze they drink, the leaner they will get. Put simply, alcohol puts the brakes on fat loss, as it interferes with the normal metabolic pathways, including fat-burning, in the body.

In addition to alcohol preventing you from burning fat, it also contributes a significant amount to your daily intake of calories. It's very easy to drink a lot of calories from alcohol without realizing it, and this can have big consequences for your training and nutrition the following day. With a hangover, you are not likely to want to train or to eat particularly well—personally, I'll eat everything in sight when hungover, including tubs and tubs of ice cream.

Ultimately you need to find your own balance, but if you really are serious about getting lean and transforming your body, then you will need to sacrifice a few nights out on the booze. Alcohol could well be the one thing holding you back from achieving the body you want.

> **" ALCOHOL PUTS THE BRAKES ON FAT LOSS "**

Hydration

. . . .

Most people underestimate the importance of hydration for fat loss. Almost two-thirds of the human body is made up of water, and it is involved in everything from removing waste and lubricating joints to regulating body temperature. It also aids metabolism, so consumption of water is vital to maximize your body's fat-burning ability. As a general rule, I recommend drinking between 2 and 4 quarts of water per day. This may seem like a lot, but it really will work wonders for your body inside and out. If you don't enjoy drinking plain water, try adding some fresh mint, lemon or lime for a bit of flavor.

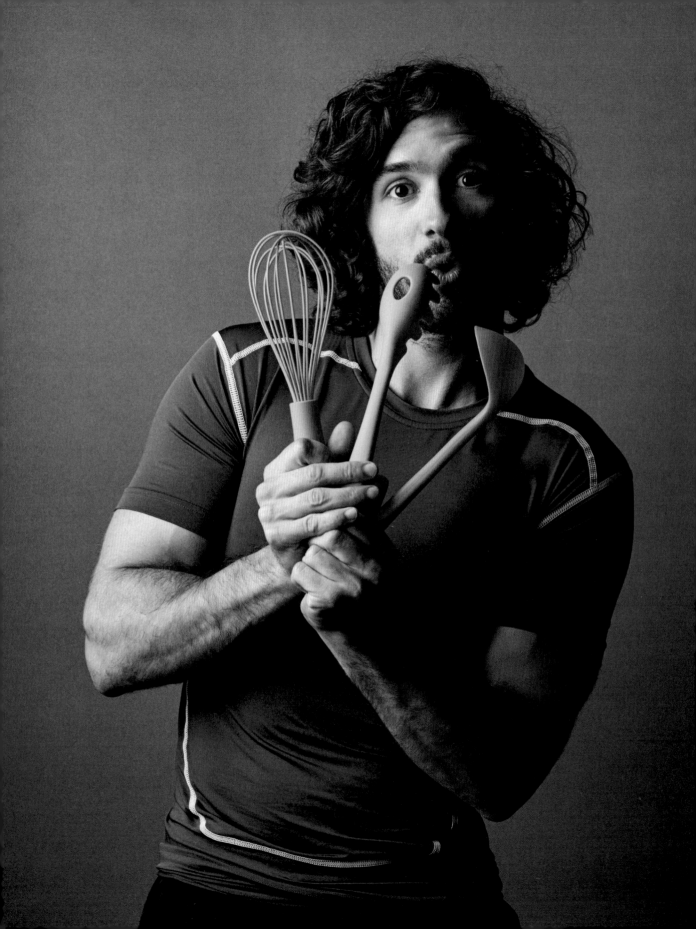

GETTING STARTED

2

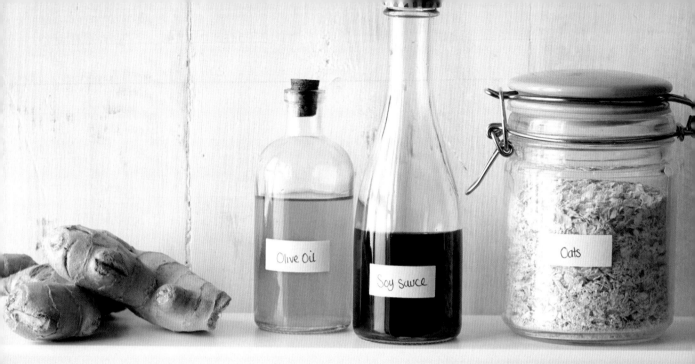

Olive Oil

Soy sauce

Oats

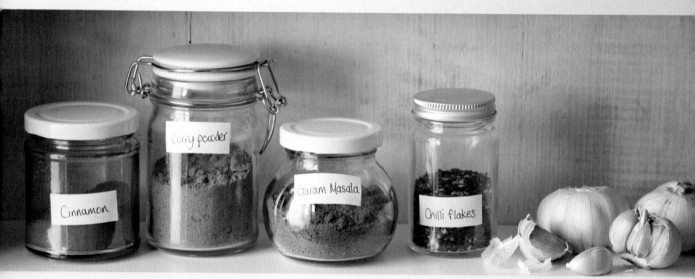

Cinnamon

Curry powder

Garam Masala

Chilli flakes

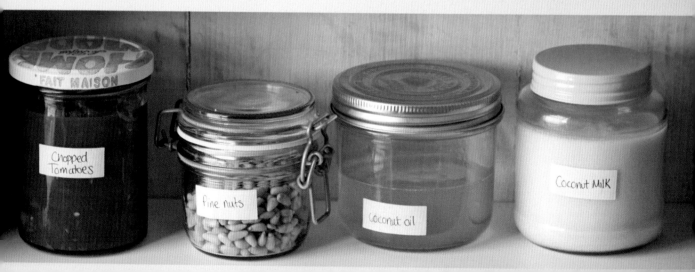

FAIT MAISON

Chopped Tomatoes

Pine nuts

Coconut oil

Coconut Milk

GETTING STARTED

///////////////////////////////////////

No more low calories, zero carbs or low fat for you

Hopefully you now have a better understanding of macro-nutrients and how you are going to use them to fuel your body to get lean. No more low calories, zero carbs or low fat for you! You are going to eat lots of tasty food, feel full of energy every day, and really give your body a chance to transform.

STEP 1:
PLAN LIKE A WINNER

Planning your meals and workouts into the week ahead is the first step for success. You may not be able to follow it 100%, as things will inevitably pop up during the week that are beyond your control. That's life, but it's still important to set yourself daily goals: if you can only manage 3 workouts per week, then that's what you should put in your plan. Keep it realistic and achievable, as small daily wins will increase your motivation to follow your plan.

Start by writing down your workouts and meals into a table like mine on page 214. This will allow you to schedule time for your workouts and also create a shopping list ready for when you prep your meals.

PREPPING LIKE A BOSS

Now you have planned like a winner it's time to get your food shopping done and get prepping like a boss. This means spending a couple of hours in the kitchen on a weekend to set yourself up for success. It may seem like a hassle to begin with, but you will get quicker and more organized, and soon it will become an easy habit for you. It's a great feeling to know exactly what you are fueling your body with, and it means you can avoid buying junk food on the go when you get hungry. You can leave the house with your lunch made and your dinner all ready to go, so that after a long day at work or a late session at the gym, you can just stroll in, reheat your meal and refuel your body quickly.

The busier your lifestyle and job are, the further in advance you will need to prep. Some people like to cook and freeze their meals for a week ahead. I personally prefer to eat a bit fresher, so I just prep my meals a day or two in advance and keep them in the fridge. I then either eat them cold or reheat them in the microwave or oven. There is no right or wrong way to do this. Just keep it as stress-free as possible and make it fit your lifestyle—that way you're more likely to stick to it and form good habits.

STEP 3:

GET STOCKED UP!

Now you know how to prep like a boss, you need a few essential tools and ingredients to start putting your plans into action:

1. Food scales—to weigh your ingredients and maintain good portion control

2. Food storage containers—to store and organize all your tasty meals for the week ahead

3. A decent wok and pan—there's nothing worse than a bad wok, so invest in a good one

4. Pantry essentials—some core ingredients in the cabinet or fridge, so you don't get caught out

> " I just prep my meals a day or two in advance and keep them in the fridge "

5. A refillable water bottle—to ensure you stay hydrated at all times and can keep track of your water intake each day

PANTRY ESSENTIALS

Garam masala
Curry powder
Fresh ginger
Ground cinnamon
Garlic
Red pepper flakes
Pine nuts
Canned tomatoes
Oats
Light soy sauce
Olive oil
Coconut oil
Coconut milk

THROW AWAY THE SAD STEP!

I call bathroom scales the sad step because that's exactly what they are: you stand on them every day, and then feel sad when the numbers aren't moving in the right direction. This often results in people losing motivation, bingeing on junk food or quitting a plan altogether. I don't want you to be concerned with the numbers anymore.

The truth is, when it comes to hitting your health and fitness goals, the sad step is the worst measure of success you can possibly get and it's time you threw it out the window. Because no matter how hard you train, or how well you eat, scales cannot measure some of the most important things when it comes to your body, health and well-being.

> **" I don't want you to be concerned with the numbers anymore "**

Things the sad step CANNOT measure:

Your fitness levels
Your energy levels
Your strength
Changes in your body composition
Your sense of achievement
Your confidence
Your happiness

The best motivational tool for measuring your progress is taking photos of your body. My advice is to take some photos at the end of each month: these will show your true progress and keep you motivated to carry on, even when the mirror starts playing tricks on you and you convince yourself you haven't changed.

GO GET LEAN

///////////////////////////////////

Once you've got your meals and workouts planned, you can start your journey to a fitter, stronger and leaner version of yourself. Remember, fat loss is a journey not a race, so be patient and be consistent.

LET'S GET SOCIAL

///////////////////////////////////

If you want to see more recipes or share your meals and progress with me, post and tag your pics with the hashtag #Leanin15 on Twitter, Instagram and Facebook @thebodycoach.

For more HIIT workouts, check out my YouTube channel TheBodyCoachTV.

> **" Fat loss is a journey not a race "**

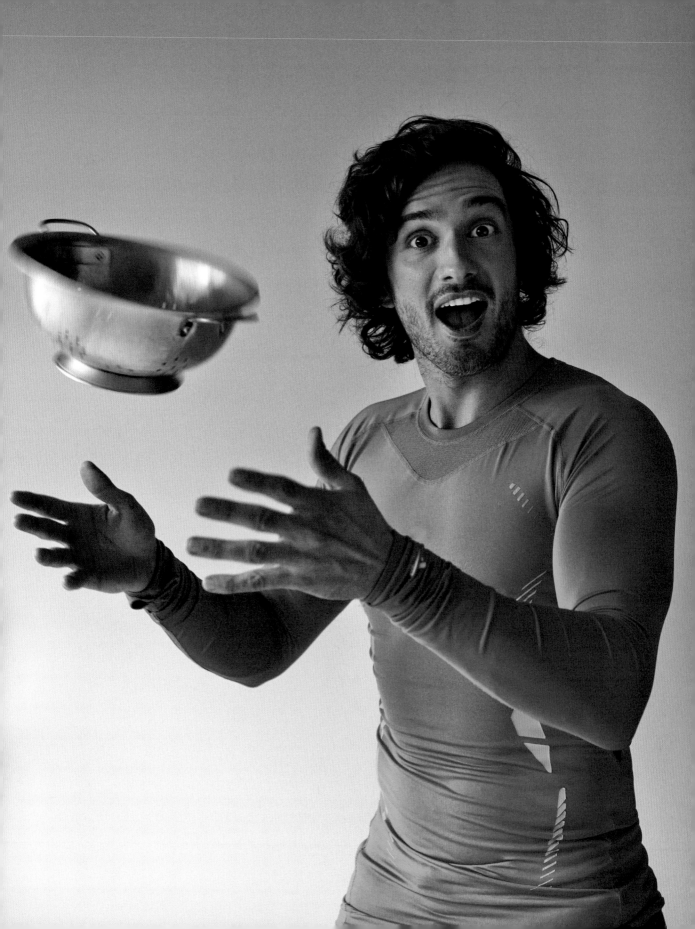

REDUCED-CARBOHYDRATE RECIPES

3

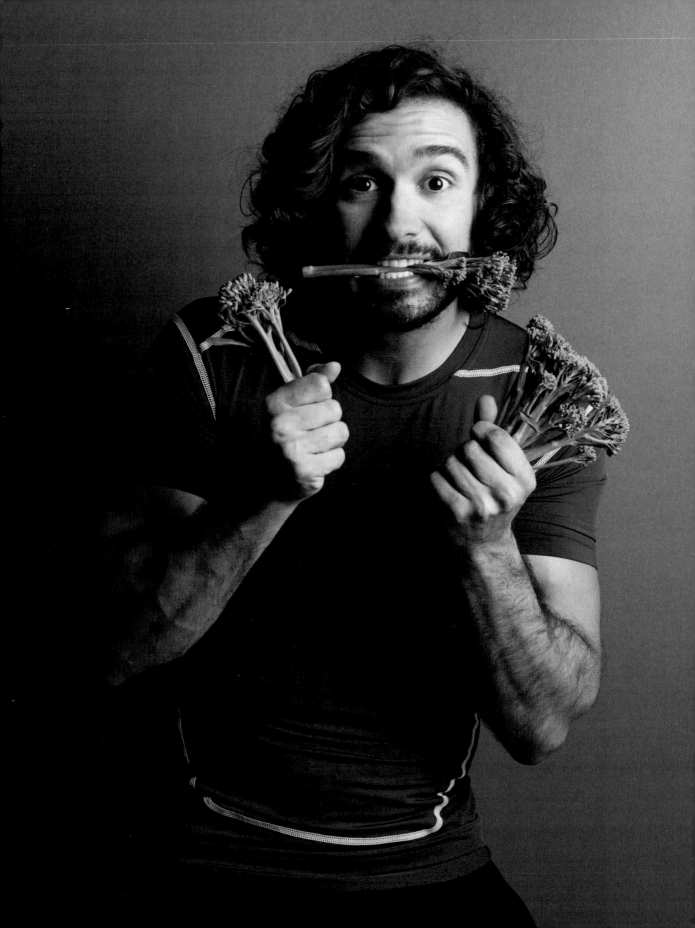

NUT AND MANGO SMOOTHIE

This fruity smoothie is ideal for a last-minute breakfast on the go. With healthy fats and a scoop of protein powder, this is way better for you than any bowl of boxed cereal. Try not to get into the habit of having smoothies every day, though. As I always say, real food wins over dust every time.

SERVES 1

INGREDIENTS

4 oz sliced mango
2 tbsp almond or cashew butter
handful of ice cubes
handful of raspberries
2 tbsp full-fat Greek yogurt
1 scoop (30g) vanilla or strawberry protein powder
½ cup almond milk

METHOD

Place all the ingredients in a blender and blend until smooth.

★ TOP TIP

Warning! Don't go nuts with your nuts. While they are a great source of protein, fiber and essential fats, nuts also contain lots of calories. It's very easy to crack open a ½-pound bag and finish the lot without feeling full. But remember every gram of fat contains 9 calories, so overeating nuts will not help with your fat loss. I recommend a snack portion of about 1 ounce. Also, try to get a variety of different nuts as they contain different vitamins. Almonds, walnuts and cashews are my personal favorites.

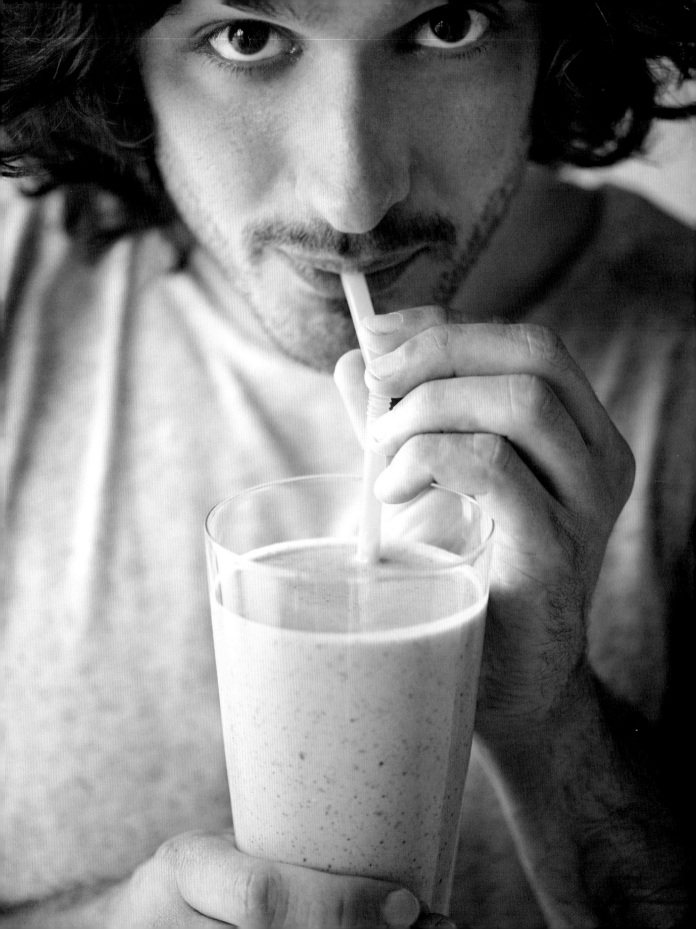

FATS-ME-UP SMOOTHIE

SERVES 1

Here's another tasty low-carb smoothie you can drink on the go. The almond milk and avocado provide you with some healthy fats for fuel, but feel free to add a scoop of your favorite protein too for an extra boost. Make sure you use a soft, ripe avocado for this.

INGREDIENTS

juice of 2 limes
1 scant cup almond milk
handful of blackberries
handful of blueberries
½ avocado, roughly chopped
3 tbsp full-fat Greek yogurt
1 tbsp honey

METHOD

Throw everything into a blender and blend until smooth.

★ TOP TIP

The avocado is a nutritional hero in my eyes, with a long list of health benefits. It's a great source of monounsaturated oleic acid, which research has shown reduces levels of bad LDL cholesterol at the same time as increasing levels of the more beneficial HDL cholesterol. That means this little rascal is actually good for your heart.

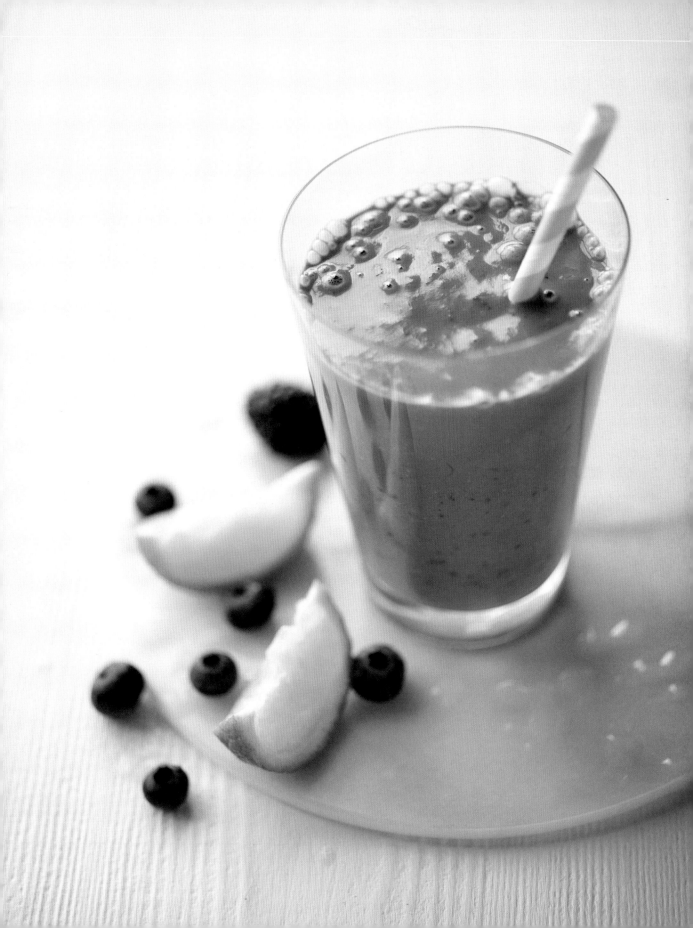

SERVES 1

INGREDIENTS

2 tbsp chia seeds

3 tbsp golden flaxseed meal

6 tbsp finely shredded unsweetened coconut

6 tbsp oats—rolled or steel-cut, not instant

¾ tsp ground cinnamon

1¼ cups almond milk, plus a little extra if needed

3 tbsp full-fat Greek yogurt

CINNAMON REDUCED-CARB OATMEAL

I always like to encourage people to think outside the cereal box at breakfast but there's nothing wrong with a good bowl of oats. The added chia and flaxseeds in this meal provide a dose of those all-important and essential omega-3 fatty acids. This one will leave you feeling full and energized until lunch.

METHOD

Place all the ingredients except the yogurt in a small saucepan and cook gently over low heat for 5–6 minutes until you're happy with the consistency—add a little more almond milk if the oatmeal gets too thick.

Transfer to a bowl, dollop the yogurt on top and serve.

★ TOP TIP

Flaxseeds (also called linseeds) are a rich source of micronutrients, dietary fiber, vitamin B1 and an omega-3 fatty acid called alpha-linoleic acid (ALA). So if you don't enjoy eating oily fish, try to get flaxseeds into your diet more often.

SERVES 1

INGREDIENTS

¾ cup coconut water

2 tbsp almond butter

1 oz fresh wheatgrass (or 5g powdered)

1 scoop (30g) vanilla protein powder

1 apple, cored and roughly chopped

2 tbsp flaxseeds

handful of baby spinach leaves

handful of ice cubes

GO-GO-GREEN SMOOTHIE

Moms always tell us to eat our greens, so here you go. If you're not a big fan of leafy green veg, then this is the perfect opportunity for you to smash them in. Wheatgrass is very good for you—but it's a love or hate kind of thing. If you don't enjoy it, just leave it out and add more spinach or some kale instead.

METHOD

Put all the ingredients in a blender and blend on high for 1 minute or until the smoothie has reached your desired texture.

CAULIFLOWER COUSCOUS CHICKEN SALAD

SERVES 2

In my opinion, cauliflower is underrated and underused. It's extremely nutritious and full of goodness. Use this recipe as a basis to experiment with other flavor combinations—try it with smoked mackerel instead of chicken, for example. If you want a warm dish, just microwave the cauliflower on its own and then add the other ingredients.

MAKE AHEAD
INGREDIENTS

1 cauliflower, broken into florets
¼ cup pomegranate seeds
5 sun-dried tomatoes, roughly chopped
2 jarred roasted red peppers, roughly chopped
2 tbsp walnut oil or olive oil
¼ cup walnuts, roughly chopped
½ bunch of chives, finely sliced
½ bunch of parsley, leaves only, roughly chopped
large handful of baby spinach leaves
¾ lb cooked skinless chicken breast (deli chicken is perfect)
juice of 1 lemon

METHOD

Place the cauliflower florets in a food processor and pulse until they have a couscous-like texture.

Tip your cauliflower couscous into a large bowl and add all the other ingredients except the chicken and lemon juice. Mix thoroughly.

Pile up your couscous on plates, then top with the cooked chicken and a good squeeze of lemon juice.

CHEESY CHORIZO CHICKEN AND SPINACH

SERVES 1

This is pretty much the simplest dish you can imagine. And melted cheese is sooooo satisfying! You can also try this with shrimp or ground turkey for a change, if you like.

INGREDIENTS

½ tbsp coconut oil
2 to 3 oz Spanish (dry-cured) chorizo, finely diced
½ red onion, diced
1 boneless, skinless chicken breast (about 8 oz), cut into ⅓-inch slices
salt and pepper
4 cherry tomatoes, sliced in half
3 big fistfuls of baby spinach leaves
1 ball of mozzarella, torn into chunks
2 tbsp pine nuts

METHOD

Heat the coconut oil in a large frying pan over medium to high heat. Add the chorizo and fry for a minute. Add the onion and fry for another minute.

Increase the heat to maximum and add the chicken, along with a generous pinch of both salt and pepper. Stir-fry for about 3 minutes, by which time the chicken should be almost completely cooked through.

Throw in the cherry tomatoes and cook for a minute or until they just begin to collapse. Toss in the spinach and stir through until fully wilted.

Use a wooden spoon to make little pockets in the chicken and vegetable mixture, then drop in small chunks of the mozzarella. Turn off the heat and let the mozzarella melt before spooning the whole delicious lot onto a plate and scattering over the pine nuts.

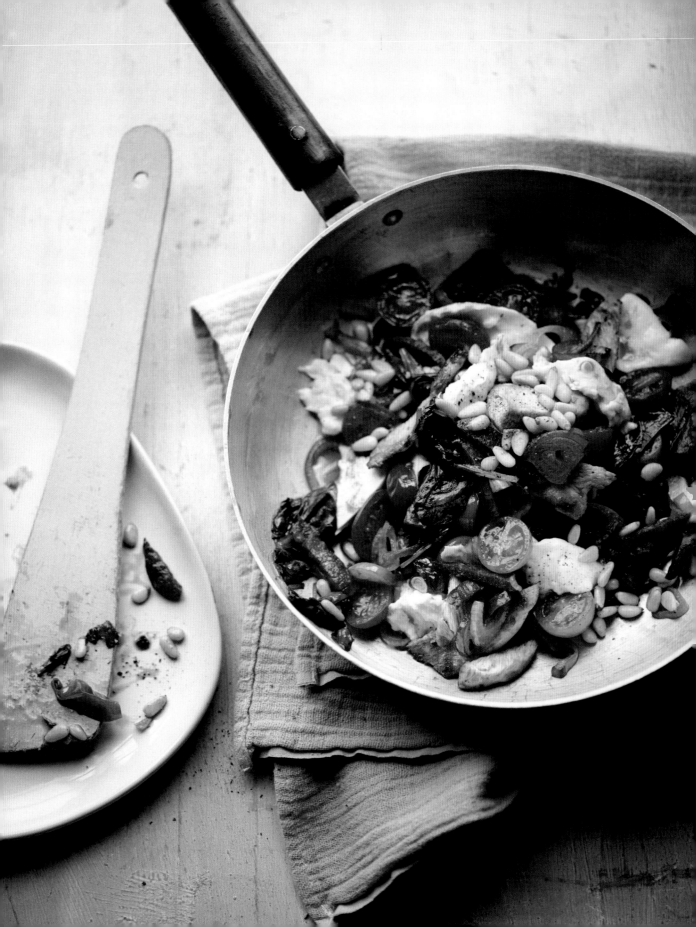

CHICKEN WITH CREAMY WILD MUSHROOM AND TARRAGON SAUCE

SERVES 2

This old-school classic really hits the spot: it's so full of flavor, and poaching the chicken keeps it nice and moist. Most supermarkets now stock some great wild mushrooms, so be adventurous and get some exotic-looking ones.

GOOD TO FREEZE
INGREDIENTS

2 boneless, skinless chicken breasts (about 8 oz each)
1 tbsp olive oil
1 clove garlic, finely chopped
10 oz mixed mushrooms—
  I like chestnut and oyster
splash of white wine
2 large handfuls of baby spinach leaves
⅔ cup heavy cream
½ bunch of tarragon, leaves only, roughly chopped
salt and pepper

METHOD

Bring a large saucepan of water to a boil, then slide in the chicken. Lower the heat until the water is just "burping" and not vigorously boiling. Let the chicken cook for 12 minutes, by which time it should be fully cooked through.

Meanwhile, heat the oil in a large frying pan over medium to high heat. Add the garlic and cook for about 30 seconds. Roughly chop any larger mushrooms and throw them into the pan, to give them a head start for a minute or two before adding the rest of the mushrooms and cooking for another minute.

Increase the heat to maximum, then pour in the white wine and let it bubble away to almost nothing. Drop in the spinach and stir until wilted. Pour in the cream, then bring to a boil and simmer for 1 minute. Add the chopped tarragon and remove the pan from the heat.

Check that the chicken is cooked by slicing into the thickest part of the breast: the meat should be white all the way through and the juices should run clear, not pink. Remove to a plate, draining off as much liquid as possible. Season with salt and pepper, then place on two plates and pour over the delicious creamy sauce.

★ Serve with a big portion of your favorite greens such as spinach, kale, broccoli, snow peas or green beans.

INGREDIENTS

**2 tsp coconut oil
2 shallots, finely sliced
5 cremini mushrooms,
   roughly chopped
10 oz filet mignon, cut into
   ⅓-inch-thick strips
salt and pepper
2 tsp smoked paprika
⅓ cup beef stock
⅔ cup sour cream
½ bunch of parsley, leaves
   only, roughly chopped—
   optional
juice of 1 lemon**

SUPER-SPEEDY BEEF STROGANOFF

Filet mignon is the best cut for this dish, but it is expensive, so if you're on a budget opt for sirloin or rump. If you love steak then this one is a real winner.

METHOD

Melt the coconut oil in a frying pan over high heat. Add the shallots and mushrooms and fry, stirring regularly, for 2–3 minutes or until the shallots have softened and the mushrooms have taken on a little color.

Add the beef, along with a generous pinch of both salt and pepper, and stir-fry for 1–2 minutes. Sprinkle in the smoked paprika and toss to lightly coat everything with the spice.

Pour in the beef stock—it will bubble up quickly—then turn the heat right down and stir in the sour cream. Take the pan off the heat, then add the parsley, if using, and a generous squeeze of lemon juice. Serve and enjoy.

★ Serve with a big portion of your favorite greens such as spinach, kale, broccoli, snow peas or green beans.

FRESH TUNA NIÇOISE

I love using fresh tuna for this salad, as it tastes amazing, but if you'd rather use canned tuna, that's fine too. This makes a great packed lunch to carry to work.

MAKE AHEAD
INGREDIENTS

1 egg
3 oz green beans, trimmed
½ tbsp coconut oil
10 oz tuna steak
salt and pepper
2 tbsp pre-cooked Puy lentils
large handful of baby
  spinach leaves
4 sun-dried tomatoes,
  roughly chopped
1 oz walnuts, roughly chopped
1 tbsp olive oil
2 tsp balsamic or sherry
  vinegar

METHOD

Bring a medium saucepan of water to a boil before carefully lowering in the egg. Boil for 8 minutes, then drop in the green beans and simmer for another minute.

Meanwhile, heat the coconut oil in a frying pan over medium to high heat. Carefully lay in the tuna and fry for 1 minute on each side. This will give you rare tuna—if you like it more cooked, fry it for another minute on each side. Remove the tuna from the pan, season and let rest while you put the rest of the salad together.

Drain the egg and beans in a sieve or colander, then run under cold water until cool enough to handle. Peel the egg and slice in half. Put the beans, lentils, spinach, sun-dried tomatoes, walnuts, olive oil and vinegar into a bowl, along with a generous pinch of salt and pepper. Gently toss all the ingredients together, then transfer to a plate.

Top the salad with the tuna, sliced if you like, and the egg.

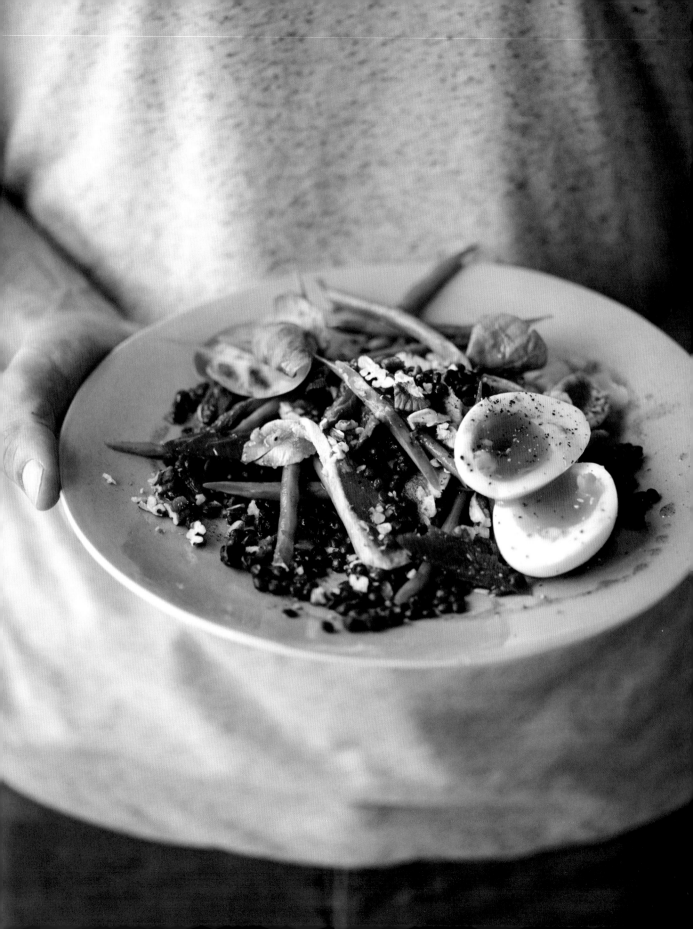

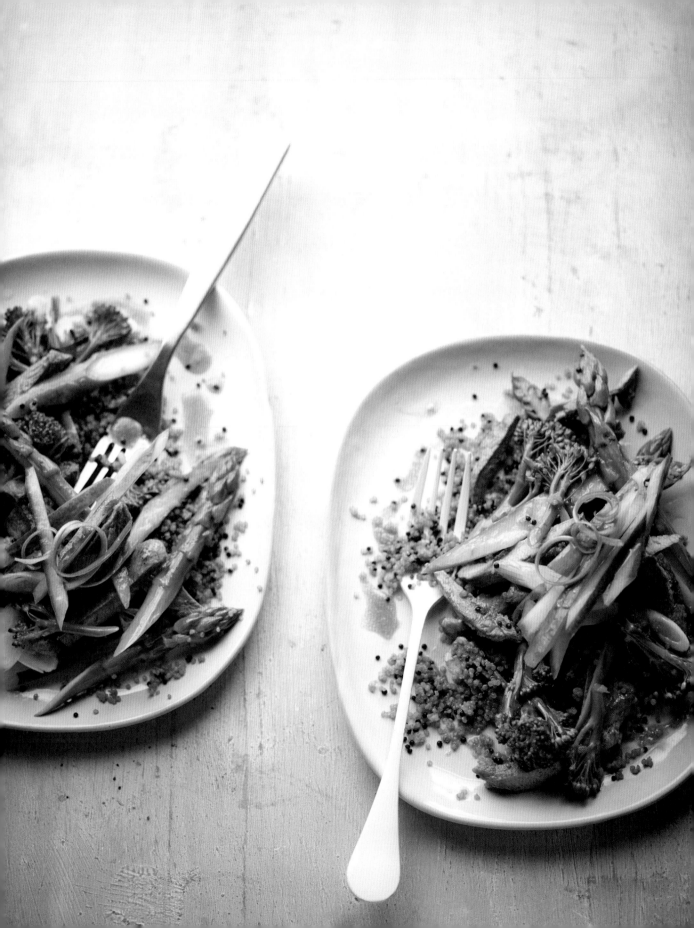

ASIAN DUCK SALAD

Duck is a rich and delicious meat that's packed with protein. For the veg, I've gone with asparagus and midget trees (my name for broccoli!), but feel free to improvise. Having fun in the kitchen and mixing it up will help to keep things tasty and vary your nutrients. As you can see, I've doubled the recipe in the picture.

MAKE AHEAD

INGREDIENTS

5 spears of asparagus
4 midget trees (broccolini), any bigger stalks sliced in half lengthwise
½ tbsp coconut oil
8 oz boneless, skinless duck breast, sliced into ⅓-inch-thick strips
¾ inch fresh ginger, finely chopped
1 tbsp light soy sauce
2 tsp sesame oil
2 tbsp pre-cooked quinoa
1 scallion, finely sliced
¼ cucumber, sliced into thin matchsticks

METHOD

Take each asparagus spear in turn and bend it gently until it snaps—it will naturally snap at the point where it becomes tender. Discard the bottom of the spear.

Bring a large saucepan of water to a boil, then drop in the asparagus and the midget trees and simmer for 1½ minutes. Drain in a sieve or colander, then rinse under cold running water.

Melt the coconut oil in a frying pan over a high heat. Add the duck and stir-fry for 30 seconds, then add the ginger and stir-fry for another minute, by which time the duck should be cooked through. Remove the pan from the heat and stir in the soy sauce and sesame oil.

Place the cooked vegetables in a bowl, then add the quinoa and the duck, along with all its juices. Mix the whole lot together before transferring to a plate and topping with the scallion and cucumber.

SERVES 4

MAKE AHEAD
GOOD TO FREEZE

INGREDIENTS

2 tbsp coconut oil

2 star anise

1 small eggplant, chopped
into small pieces

2 tbsp Thai green curry paste,
homemade (see Top Tip) or
store-bought

1 can (13.5 oz) full-fat
coconut milk

handful of baby corn

1 lb raw jumbo shrimp, peeled

1–2 tbsp fish sauce

3 limes

½ bunch of basil, leaves only,
roughly chopped

½ bunch of cilantro, leaves
only, roughly chopped

1 red chile, roughly chopped—
remove the seeds if you
don't like it hot

THAI GREEN CURRY

This tasty classic is my all-time favorite meal. In this version I've suggested shrimp, but chicken and pork would work just as well. Bump up the flavor by using full-fat coconut milk, which is packed with good fat. Fish sauce is great to have in the pantry: it keeps for ages, and even though it smells terrible, it tastes amazing.

METHOD

Melt the coconut oil in a large saucepan over medium to high heat. Add the star anise and eggplant and fry for 1 minute, then add in the curry paste and half the coconut milk. Stir the paste into the milk, then increase the heat to maximum.

Pour in the rest of the coconut milk, then half-fill the can with water, slosh it around and pour this into the pan as well. Toss in the corn, then bring to a boil and simmer for 3 minutes. Drop in the shrimp and simmer for another 2 minutes until they turn pink and are fully cooked.

Take the pan off the heat and add the fish sauce to taste, the juice of 2 of the limes, the herbs and the chile.

Serve up the curry in bowls, with the last lime cut into quarters for squeezing.

★ **TOP TIP**

Here's my recipe to make your own Thai green curry paste:

4 banana shallots, peeled and
chopped

1½ inches fresh galangal, peeled
and chopped

4 cloves garlic, peeled and
chopped

2 stalks lemongrass, trimmed
and chopped

1 tsp cumin seeds

½ tsp coriander seeds

1 bunch of basil

2 bunches of cilantro

1 tbsp fish sauce

pinch of grated star anise

Blend everything together using either a little warm water or coconut milk to loosen. You can keep this in an airtight container in the fridge for up to 5 days.

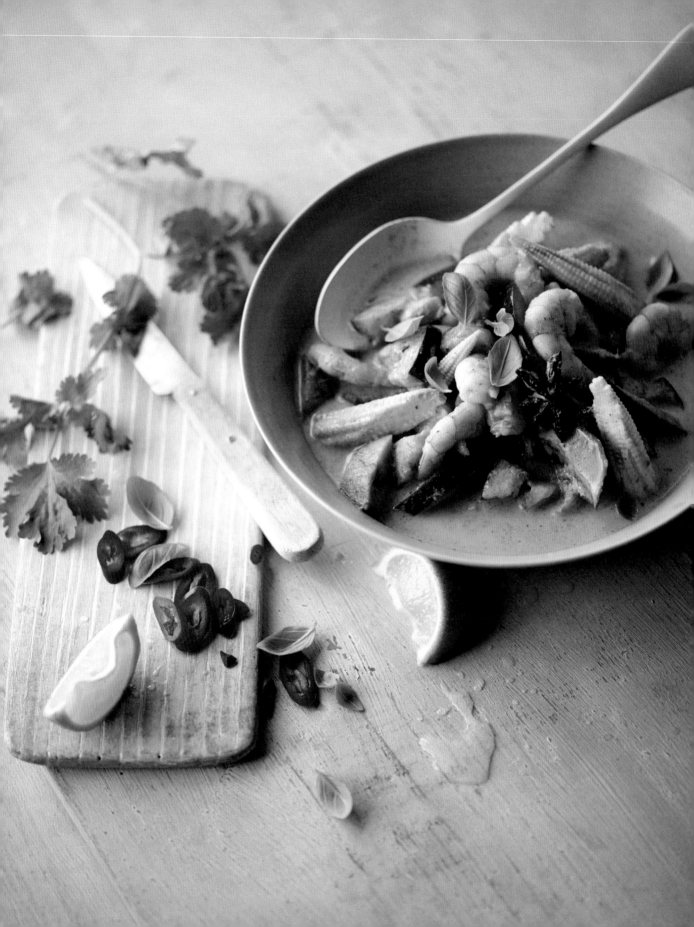

MAKE AHEAD
GOOD TO FREEZE
INGREDIENTS

4 tsp butter
2 slices Canadian bacon,
   cut into ⅓-inch strips
½ red onion, diced
1 clove garlic, finely chopped
½ lb cod fillet, skinned and
   cut into ¾-inch chunks
1 can (14 oz) chopped
   tomatoes
8 pitted black olives
1 ball of mozzarella, torn
   into chunks
2 tbsp pine nuts
basil leaves, to serve—
   optional

FRENCH-STYLE COD WITH BLACK OLIVES

This is a simple and delicious dish based on a classic French combo. If you're not a fan of cod, you could use any other white fish of your choice.

METHOD

Melt the butter in a large frying pan over medium to high heat. Add the bacon and onion and fry for 2 minutes or until the onion is starting to soften and the bacon is cooked. Add the garlic and cook for another 30 seconds.

Drop in the chunks of cod and fry, turning the chunks every now and then, for 2 minutes. Add the tomatoes and bring to boil. Reduce the heat to a simmer and cook for 2–3 minutes.

Add the olives and mozzarella, then take the pan off the heat and let the mozzarella melt in the residual heat.

Serve the cod topped with the pine nuts—and the basil leaves, if using.

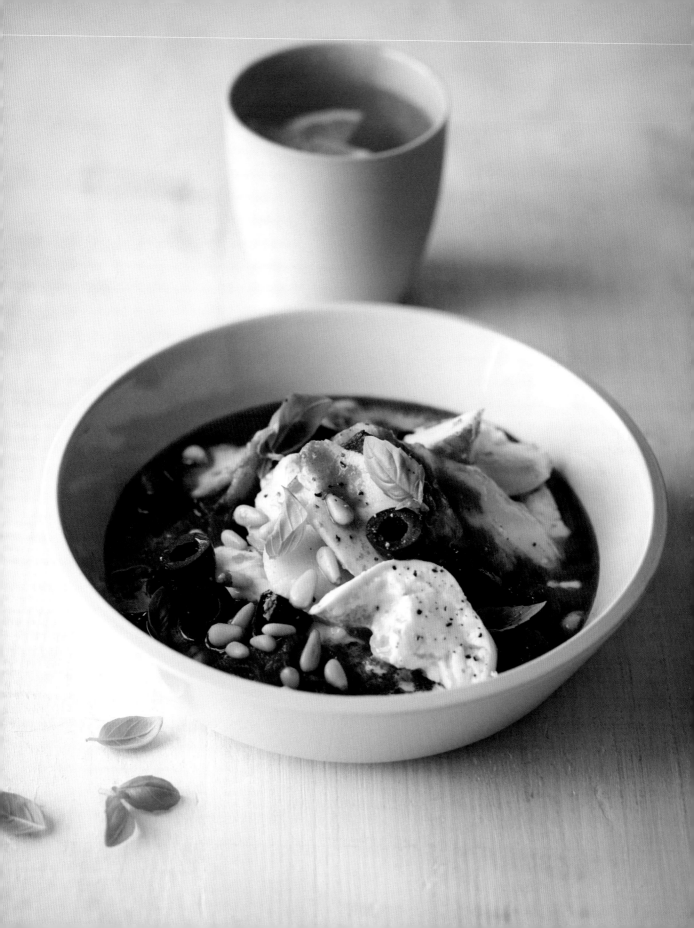

EGGS BAKED IN AVOCADO

This is becoming a bit of a signature dish for me. I've posted it a few times, and I love seeing people make it at home and share it on Instagram. It contains more healthy fats than you can shake a stick at . . . oh, and it's got bacon too, so you know it's going to taste as good as it looks.

INGREDIENTS

4 slices Canadian bacon
1 ripe avocado
2 eggs
salt and pepper
1 red chile, finely sliced—
  remove the seeds if you
  don't like it hot

METHOD

Preheat the broiler to high, then lay the bacon on the broiler pan or a baking sheet and slide underneath. Broil for 3 minutes on each side.

Meanwhile, cut your avocado in half, remove the pit and scoop out a generous tablespoon of flesh from each half to create a hole big enough for the egg. No need to waste the leftover avocado—you can save it to make some guacamole or just eat it on the spot!

Crack an egg into each avocado half, season with a little salt and pepper and place on a microwaveable plate. Microwave the eggs in 30-second bursts for 2 minutes—this should ensure firm whites, but runny yolks.

Serve up the baked eggs and avocado with the bacon and a scattering of chile.

★ TOP TIP

To stop the avocados rocking on the plate, slice off a little bit underneath to make a flat base.

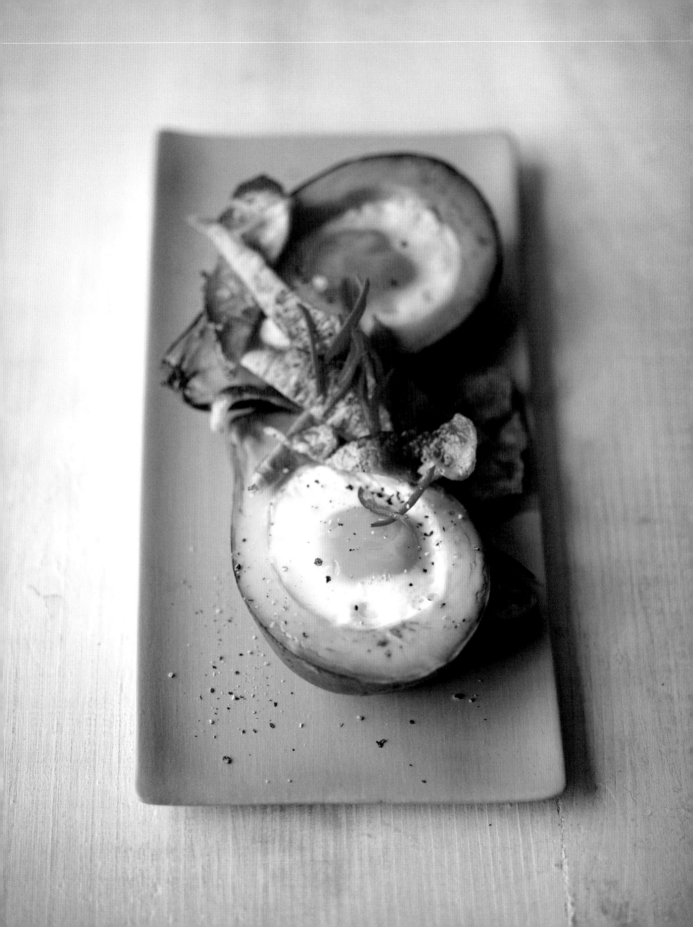

INDIAN SPICED LAMB

This is proper dinner-party food! You can see I've doubled the recipe in the picture. Make sure you buy cutlets not chops, because they have a better meat-to-fat ratio. And if you have any leftovers (not likely!), they are delicious the next day, served at room temperature with a big salad.

SERVES 1

MAKE AHEAD
INGREDIENTS

⅔ cup plain yogurt
2 tbsp ground almonds
2 tsp garam masala
1 tsp smoked paprika
salt and pepper
4 lamb cutlets (about
   7 oz each)
large handful of baby
   spinach leaves
4 cherry tomatoes, halved
¼ cucumber, sliced into
   matchsticks
½ bunch of cilantro, leaves
   only, roughly chopped
juice of 1 lemon

METHOD

Preheat the broiler to high and line a baking sheet with parchment paper (this is just to make cleanup easier).

Place the yogurt, ground almonds, garam masala and smoked paprika in a bowl, along with a generous amount of salt and pepper. Mix thoroughly.

Smother the lamb cutlets with the spiced yogurt, then place on the prepared baking sheet. Slide under the broiler and cook the cutlets for 3–4 minutes on each side, by which time the spiced yogurt should have browned in a few places.

Meanwhile, make a quick salad by gently tossing the spinach, tomatoes and cucumber together in a bowl. Pile the salad onto a plate.

Remove the lamb cutlets from the broiler and let rest for 1 or 2 minutes, then sit them on top of the salad. Serve up with a scattering of cilantro and a squeeze of lemon juice.

★ Serve with a big portion of your favorite greens such as kale, broccoli, snow peas or green beans.

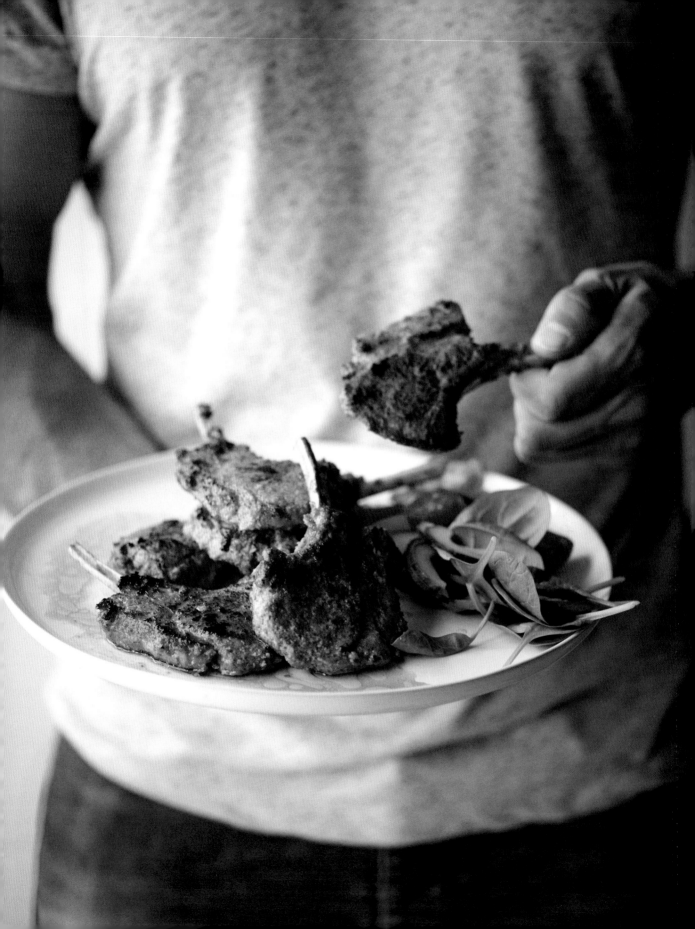

MAKE AHEAD

INGREDIENTS

½ tbsp coconut oil
½ red onion, finely chopped
1 clove garlic, finely chopped
1 red bell pepper, sliced
2 tsp smoked paprika
1 tsp dried oregano
1 boneless, skinless chicken
  breast (about 8 oz), sliced
  into ⅓-inch-thick strips
5 cherry tomatoes, cut in half
2 tbsp blanched almonds
large handful of baby
  spinach leaves
salt and pepper
juice of 1 lemon

CHICKEN WITH SMOKED PAPRIKA AND ALMONDS

This is Spanish cooking at its best. I love the combo of almonds and paprika! It's really tasty and so easy to make.

METHOD

Melt the coconut oil in a large frying pan over medium to high heat. Add the onion, garlic and bell pepper and fry, stirring regularly, for 2 minutes or until the vegetables are just starting to soften.

Sprinkle in the smoked paprika and oregano and stir to coat the vegetables, then increase the heat to high. Add the chicken and tomatoes and cook, still stirring regularly, for 3–4 minutes or until the chicken is fully cooked through. Check by slicing into one of the larger pieces to make sure the meat is white all the way through, with no raw pink bits left.

Stir in the almonds and spinach, then cook for another 2 minutes, or until the spinach has totally wilted.

Plate up your chicken, season generously with salt and pepper, and finish with a squeeze of lemon juice.

★ Serve with a big portion of your favorite greens such as spinach, kale, broccoli, snow peas or green beans.

SALMON WITH CHILE EDAMAME

Edamame (green soy beans) are now available already shelled and frozen, so take advantage of them! This salad is high in omega-3 fatty acids to keep you lean and healthy—and it makes a perfect packed lunch.

MAKE AHEAD

INGREDIENTS

1 skin-on salmon fillet (about 8 oz)

7 oz frozen edamame

1 red chile, finely diced— remove the seeds if you don't like it hot

1 tsp honey

2 tsp fish sauce

1 tbsp light soy sauce

2 tsp sesame oil

2 scallions, finely sliced

1 red bell pepper, sliced

¼ cup walnuts

handful of arugula leaves

METHOD

Bring two saucepans of water to a boil, then slide the salmon fillet into one and drop the edamame into the other. Simmer the edamame for 1½ minutes, then drain in a sieve or colander and rinse under cold running water. Poach the salmon for 12 minutes, or until just cooked through. Using a slotted spoon, carefully lift out the fish and place on a plate. When it is cool enough to handle, peel off the skin.

Meanwhile, mix together the chile, honey, fish sauce, soy sauce, sesame oil and scallions to make a dressing.

Tip the edamame into a bowl and add the bell pepper, walnuts and arugula. Pour over the dressing and toss together.

Place the salad on a plate and serve the salmon on top. This tastes great still warm from the cooking or at room temperature—you decide!

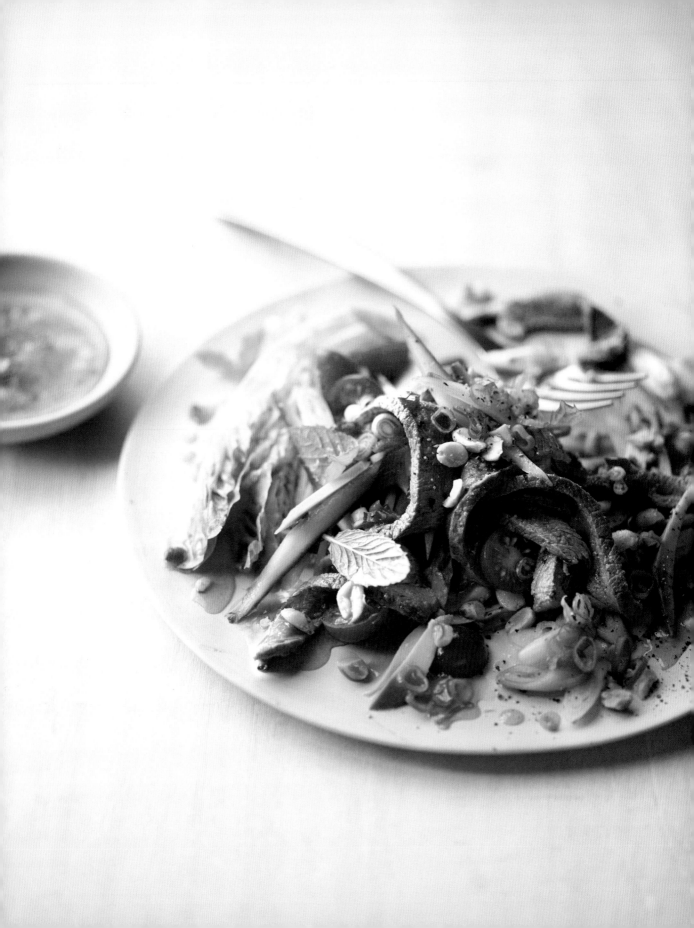

SERVES 1

THAI BEEF SALAD

This is also fantastic with shrimp or chicken instead of the beef. You can make up a big batch of the dressing and keep it in the fridge for up to 3 days.

MAKE AHEAD

INGREDIENTS

½ tbsp coconut oil

½ lb sirloin steak, trimmed of visible fat

salt and pepper

1 tbsp fish sauce

juice of 2 limes

1 lemongrass stalk, tender white part only, finely sliced

1 red chile, finely sliced— remove the seeds if you don't like it hot

2 tsp sesame oil

¼ cucumber, sliced into thin matchsticks

2 scallions, finely sliced

1 avocado, finely sliced

4 cherry tomatoes, cut in half

1 baby gem lettuce, leaves separated

2 tbsp peanuts, roughly chopped

mint and cilantro leaves, to serve

METHOD

Heat the coconut oil in a frying pan over high heat. Season the steak all over with salt and pepper. When the oil has melted and is hot, carefully lay the steak in the pan and fry for 2 minutes on each side. When the steak has had its time, transfer it to a plate and let rest for 2 minutes.

While the steak is cooking, make a dressing by mixing together the fish sauce, lime juice, lemongrass, chile and sesame oil in a large bowl. Stir in the cucumber and scallions, then let sit for 2 minutes.

When you are ready to eat, add the avocado, tomatoes and lettuce to the bowl with the dressing, cucumber and scallions, and gently toss together.

Pile up your salad on a plate, slice your steak and place lovingly on the salad, before finishing with the chopped peanuts and roughly torn cilantro and mint.

TUNA STEAK WITH SALSA

If you're not a fan of canned tuna, then get your hands on a fresh tuna steak. This sort of meal is as good for you as it tastes: the tuna is stacked with protein, and the avocado fuels your body with the healthy fats it needs.

INGREDIENTS

10 oz tuna steak
salt and pepper
1 tbsp coconut oil
2 scallions, finely sliced
2 tbsp canned black-eyed
  peas
1 avocado, roughly diced
½ mango (about 4 oz),
  roughly diced
1 small tomato, roughly diced
1 tbsp olive oil
juice of 1 lime
¼ bunch of cilantro, leaves
  only, roughly chopped

METHOD

Season the tuna generously with salt and pepper. Melt the oil in a frying pan or griddle pan over high heat. Gently lay the tuna in the pan and cook for about 2 minutes on each side, or until it's done to your liking. Be careful not to overcook it, as tuna is lean and dries out easily. Transfer the tuna to a plate and let rest while you prepare the salsa.

To make the salsa, simply mix together all the remaining ingredients and taste for seasoning.

Spoon the salsa over your perfect tuna steak.

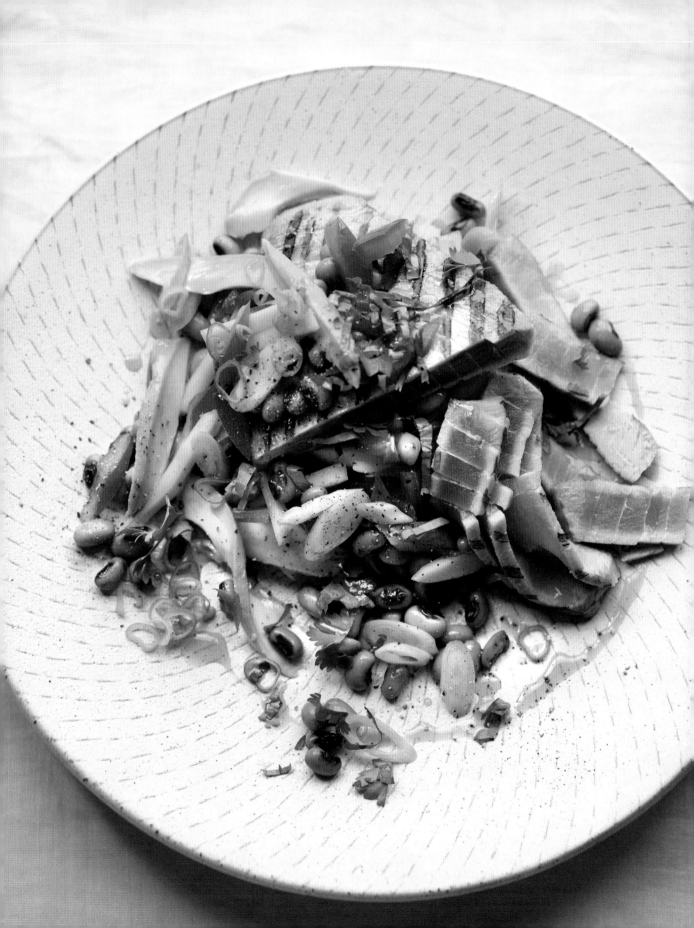

MAKE AHEAD
GOOD TO FREEZE
(only the ratatouille, not the fish)
INGREDIENTS

- **1 tbsp coconut oil**
- **1 small red onion, roughly diced**
- **1 small zucchini, cut into ⅓-inch pieces**
- **1 small eggplant, cut into ⅓-inch pieces**
- **1 sprig of thyme**
- **1 tbsp tomato paste**
- **2 tsp balsamic vinegar**
- **2 skinless salmon fillets (about 8 oz each)**

QUICK POACHED SALMON WITH SPEEDY RAT-A-TAT-A-TOUILLE

Ratatouille doesn't have to take ages! Just make sure you chop all the vegetables to roughly the same, small size, so they cook quickly and evenly.

METHOD

Bring a large saucepan of water to a boil, ready to poach the salmon.

Meanwhile, melt the coconut oil in a large saucepan over medium to high heat. Add the onion, zucchini and eggplant and stir-fry for about 4 minutes or until they are just starting to soften and color.

Drop in the thyme and stir for another minute, then add the tomato paste and mix to coat the vegetables. Keep frying, stirring continuously, for about 45 seconds before pouring in the balsamic vinegar and ½ cup of water. Bring to a boil, then reduce to a simmer and let the ratatouille bubble away for about 10 minutes, or just until the vegetables are soft. If it seems to be getting too thick, add another ¼ cup or so of water.

While the veggies are simmering away, slide the salmon fillets into the boiling water. Bring back to a simmer, then cook the fish for 10 minutes, or until just cooked through.

Using a slotted spoon, carefully lift the fish out of the water and drain well. Serve up your yummy ratatouille topped with the juicy salmon.

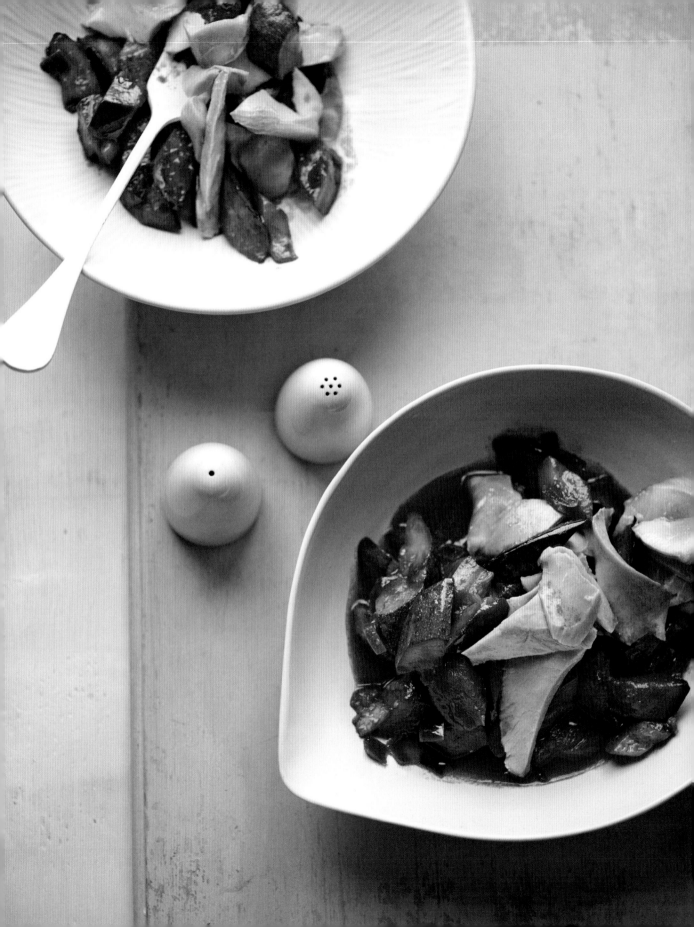

GROUND TURKEY LETTUCE BOATS

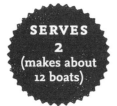

SERVES 2
(makes about 12 boats)

Spicy, fiery and packed with flavor, these little boats work as well for a dinner party as they do for a quick lunch. If you're bored of ground turkey, try making these with ground beef or shrimp instead.

MAKE AHEAD

INGREDIENTS

1 tbsp coconut oil
1 lb ground turkey
5 scallions, finely sliced
2 cloves garlic, finely chopped
1 red chile, finely sliced— remove the seeds if you don't like it hot
1 tbsp fish sauce
juice of 1 lime
small bunch of cilantro, leaves only, roughly chopped
2 avocados, roughly chopped
2 tomatoes, roughly chopped
2–3 baby gem lettuces, leaves separated

METHOD

Heat the coconut oil in a large frying pan over high heat. Add the turkey and fry for 2–3 minutes, breaking up the meat as you cook. Add the scallions, garlic and chile and stir-fry for another 2 minutes, by which time the turkey should be cooked through. Add the fish sauce, lime juice and cilantro. Mix everything together well, then remove the pan from the heat.

Combine the avocados and tomatoes in a bowl.

Lay out the lettuce leaves like little boats on your serving plate, then spoon in the turkey mixture and top with the avocados and tomatoes. Now go to munchies town and enjoy.

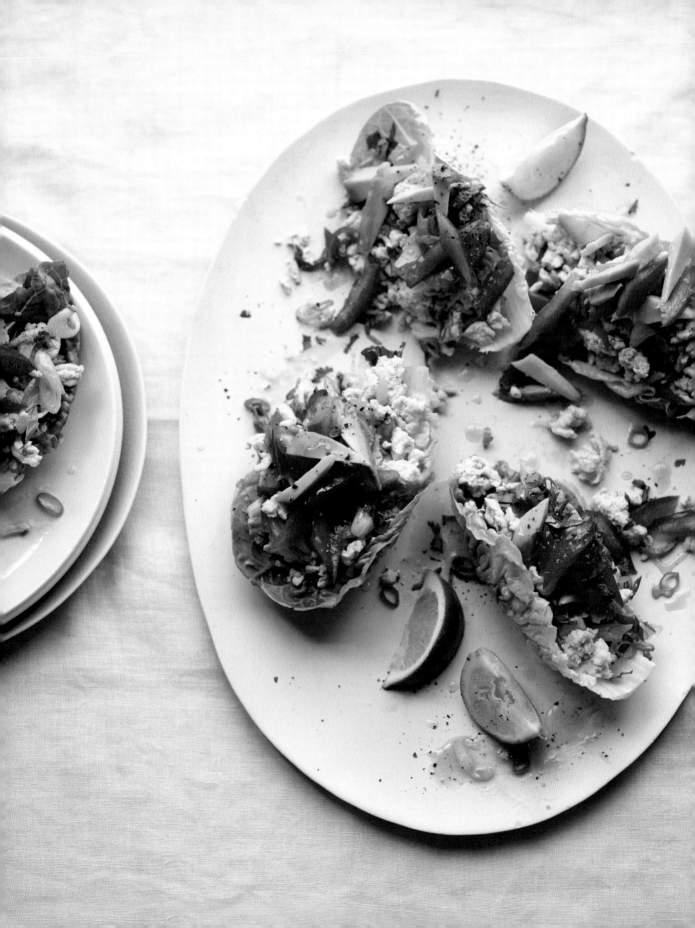

ITALIAN STALLION SAUSAGES

SERVES 2

MAKE AHEAD
GOOD TO FREEZE
INGREDIENTS

- **4 Italian sausages**
- **1 tbsp olive oil**
- **1 tsp fennel seeds**
- **2 shallots, roughly diced**
- **1 clove garlic, roughly chopped**
- **1 sprig of thyme**
- **2 fennel bulbs, roughly diced**
- **2 celery stalks, roughly diced**
- **1 zucchini, roughly diced**
- **6 cherry tomatoes**
- **1 tbsp tomato paste**
- **1 cup chicken stock**
- **½ bunch of parsley, leaves only, roughly chopped**

Oooh, if you love a bit of sausage, then this one's for you. It requires a few more ingredients than most of my Lean in 15 meals, but it's well worth the extra effort. This makes enough for two—or a meal for one, with the leftovers boxed up for the next day.

METHOD

Preheat the broiler to high. Arrange the sausages on a broiler pan and cook for 11 to 12 minutes, turning them halfway through, or until well browned and cooked through. Check by slicing into one of the sausages to make sure there are no raw pink bits left.

While the sausages are cooking, heat the oil in a large saucepan and fry the fennel seeds for about 20 seconds until they smell toasty. Add the shallots, garlic, thyme, fennel, celery and zucchini and stir-fry for 2 minutes or until just starting to soften. Add the tomatoes and the tomato paste and keep stirring for another minute.

Pour in the chicken stock and bring to boil, then reduce to a simmer. Slip the cooked sausages into the pan and let it bubble away for a minute. Stir in the parsley, then dish up.

★ Serve with a big portion of your favorite greens such as spinach, kale, broccoli, snow peas or green beans.

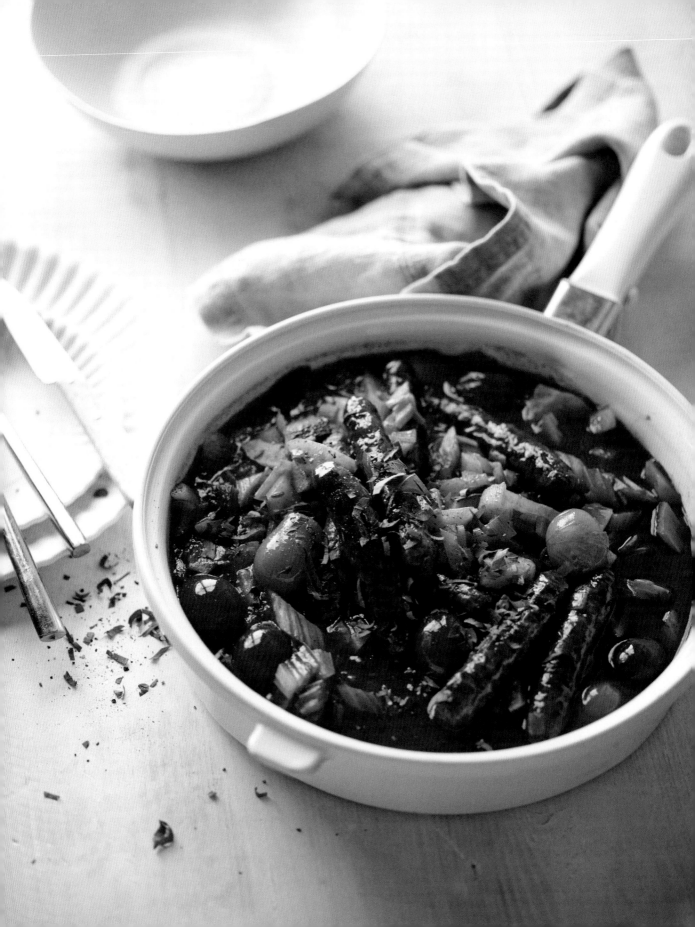

CREAMY STEAK AND SPINACH

SERVES 2

OMG—steak, wine and heavy cream? Am I dreaming?
It feels naughty, but you'll love the taste of this one, and it's
packed with healthy fats and protein.

INGREDIENTS

2 tbsp olive oil
2 sirloin steaks (8 to
   10 oz each), trimmed
   of visible fat
salt and pepper
8 mushrooms, roughly
   chopped
splash of white wine
4 large handfuls of baby
   spinach leaves
⅓ cup heavy cream

METHOD

Heat a frying pan over high heat. Drizzle 1 tablespoon of
the olive oil over the steaks, rubbing it into the flesh, and
season all over with salt and pepper. Lay the steaks in the hot
frying pan and cook for 3 minutes on each side. This will give
you medium-rare steak—if you prefer your meat medium or
well done, increase the time until it's cooked to your liking.
When you are happy with your steak, remove it from the
frying pan and let it rest on a plate while you make your
creamy side dish.

Wipe out the frying pan with paper towels, pour in the
remaining olive oil and place over medium to high heat.
Add the mushrooms and cook, flipping them a couple of
times, for 1–2 minutes or until lightly colored. Season with
salt and pepper and crank the heat up to maximum.

Pour in the white wine and let it bubble away to almost
nothing. Add the spinach and gently turn it in the pan until
it is almost fully wilted. Pour in the cream and let it bubble up.
Check the seasoning and add more salt and pepper if needed.

Take a minute to look at what a delicious meal you've made,
before wolfing it down!

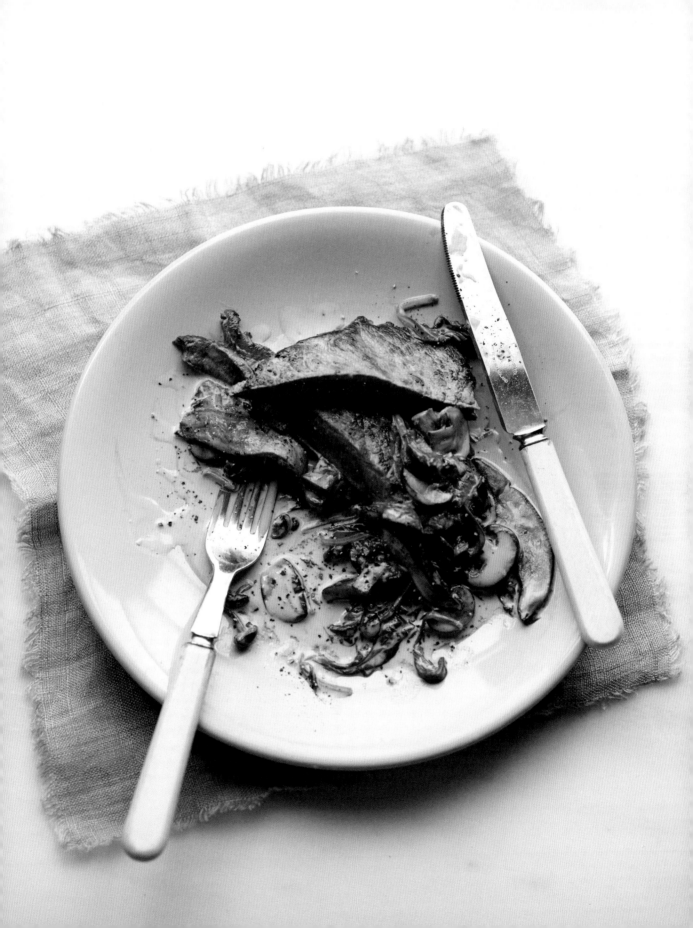

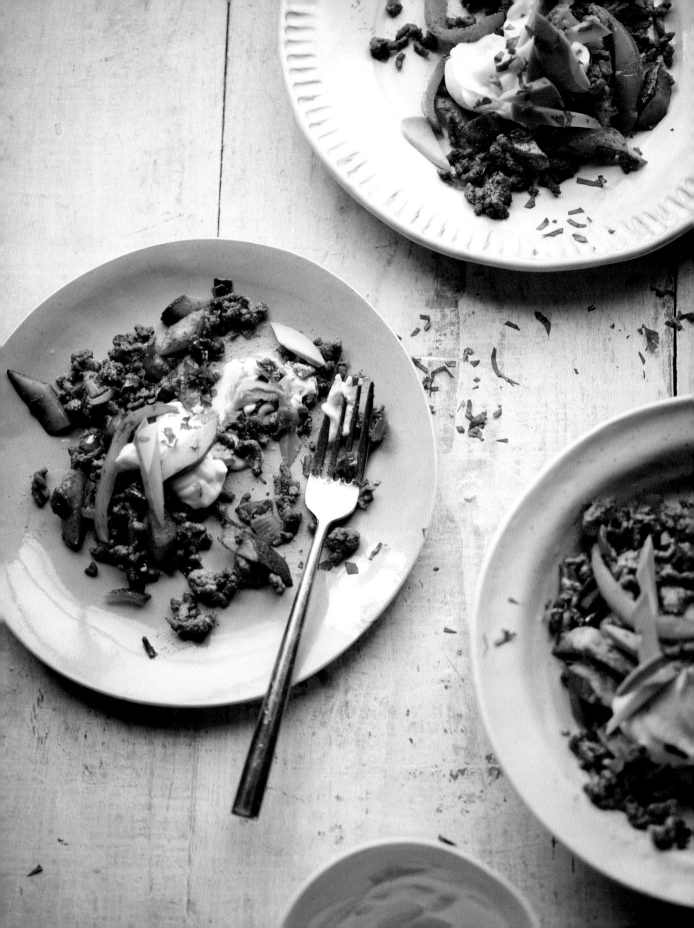

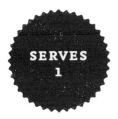

CHILI CON AVOCADO

This is a "chuck everything in the pan" kinda dish: super-simple and tasty! It tastes great cold too, perfect for a packed lunch.

MAKE AHEAD
INGREDIENTS

½ tbsp coconut oil

1 small red onion, diced

1 green chile, finely chopped—remove the seeds if you don't like it hot

1 red or yellow bell pepper, sliced

½ zucchini, diced

10 oz 95% lean ground beef

1 tsp smoked paprika

2 tsp ground cumin

salt and pepper

1 tbsp full-fat Greek yogurt

½ avocado, sliced

½ bunch of cilantro, leaves only, roughly chopped— optional

METHOD

Heat the coconut oil in a large frying pan over high heat. Add the onion, chile, bell pepper and zucchini and stir-fry for 1–2 minutes or until the vegetables start to soften and color.

Add the beef and stir to combine with the other ingredients, using your spoon to break up any large lumps as you go. Keep frying for about 3 minutes, by which time the beef should be fully cooked through.

Add the paprika and cumin, along with a generous pinch of salt and pepper, and cook for 30 seconds more.

Tip out your chili onto a plate, then top with the yogurt, avocado and cilantro, if using, and serve.

GOAN FISH CURRY

You don't need to go to India to enjoy a good curry. This recipe is surprisingly easy, but tastes incredible. If you're not fond of fish, you could always use ½ pound of boneless, skinless chicken breast instead. This is a good meal to batch-cook and freeze when you're prepping like a boss . . .

MAKE AHEAD
GOOD TO FREEZE

INGREDIENTS

3 cloves garlic, roughly chopped
1¼ inches fresh ginger, roughly chopped
1 green chile, roughly chopped—remove the seeds if you don't like it hot
2 tomatoes, roughly chopped
1 tbsp coconut oil
1 red onion, diced
1 tbsp garam masala
1 tbsp ground cumin
1 can (13.5 oz) full-fat coconut milk
1 lb haddock fillet, skinned and cut into large chunks
juice of 1 lime
½ bunch of cilantro, leaves only, roughly chopped

METHOD

Puree the garlic, ginger, chile and tomatoes in a food processor until smooth, then set aside.

Melt the oil in a wok or large frying pan over medium to high heat. Throw in the onion and fry for 2 minutes, stirring regularly. Sprinkle in the garam masala and cumin and fry, stirring continuously, for 30 seconds. Pour in the pureed ingredients and bring to a boil before pouring in the coconut milk. Return to a boil again, then let it simmer for 2 minutes.

Add the haddock pieces to the curry, and bring back to a simmer. Cook the fish for about 3 minutes, or until it is just cooked through.

Stir in the lime juice and cilantro, then serve.

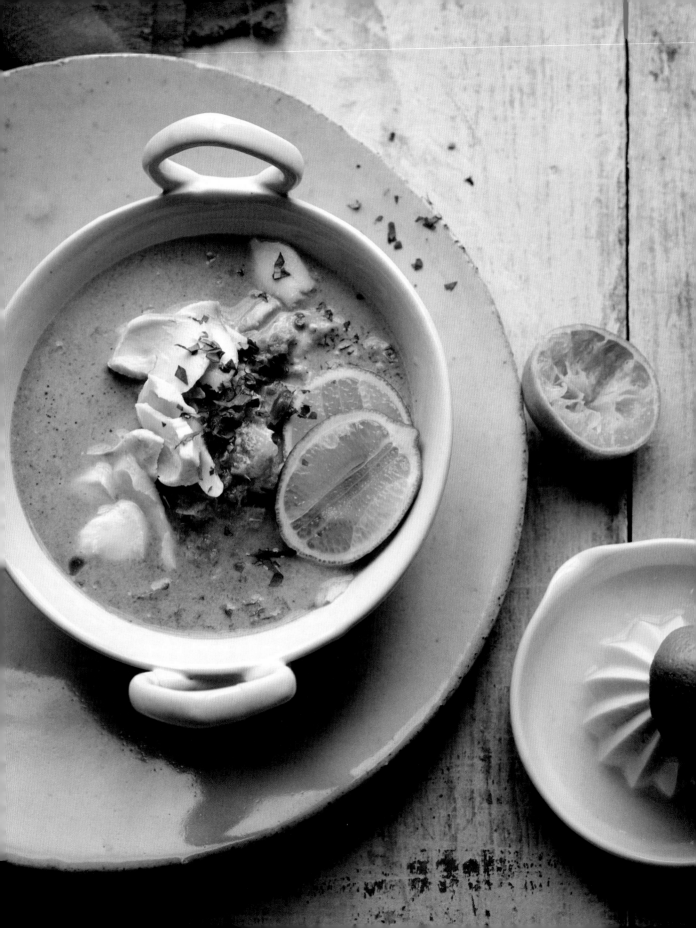

TOMATOES, EGGS AND CHORIZO

SERVES 1

If you love chorizo, this is perfect for you. Frying the chorizo with the tomatoes brings out all of the delicious flavor, and the eggs provide a dose of healthy fats.

INGREDIENTS

½ tbsp olive oil
3 oz chorizo (the cured type, not the softer fresh chorizo), chopped
pinch of red pepper flakes
2 scallions, finely sliced
1 can (14 oz) of chopped tomatoes
2 eggs
2 tbsp finely grated parmesan
sprinkling of chopped parsley, if you're feeling fancy

METHOD

Heat the oil in a small frying pan. Add the chorizo, pepper flakes and scallions and fry for about 2 minutes, stirring regularly.

Pour in the tomatoes and bring to a boil, then simmer for 1 minute. Reduce the heat to medium to low and use the back of a spoon to fashion two dips in the tomatoes as best you can. Crack an egg into each dip, sprinkle the parmesan over the eggs and place a lid on top (if you don't have a lid for your pan, a big dinner plate or a sheet of foil should work). Simmer for 5–6 minutes or until the whites are cooked, but the yolks are still runny.

Sprinkle with chopped parsley, if you like, then gobble it up straight from the pan.

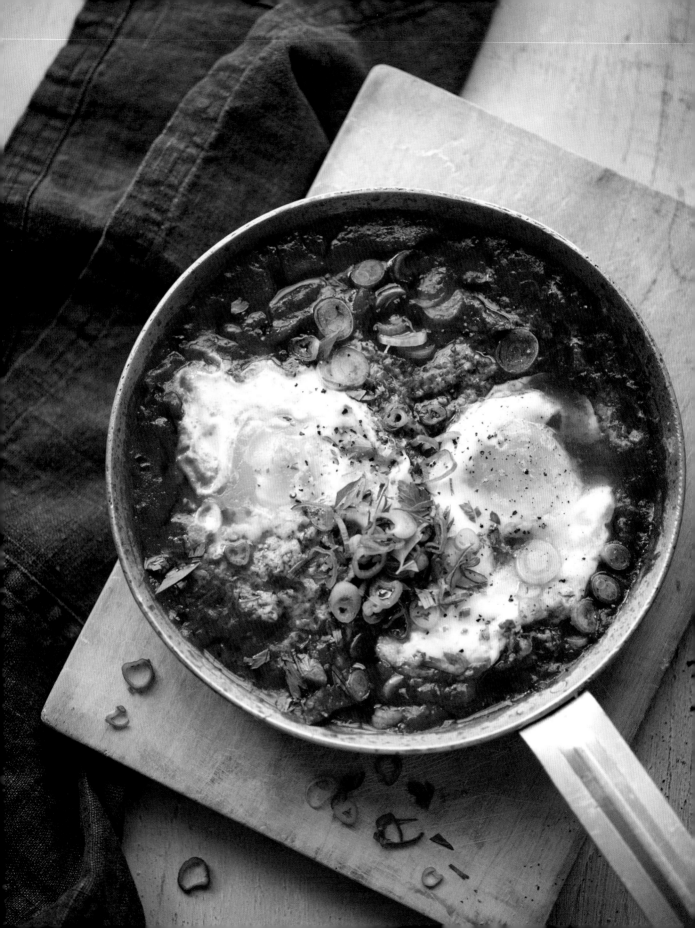

SHRIMP AND BEAN SPROUT OMELET

This is my version of Egg Foo Yung, and it's a really quick breakfast option. Feel free to add other vegetables to the mix too.

INGREDIENTS

3 eggs
2 tsp light soy sauce
2 tsp toasted sesame oil
pepper
1 tbsp peanut oil
7 oz cooked shrimp
1 oz bean sprouts
½ red chile, finely sliced—
  remove the seeds if you
  don't like it hot
2 tbsp cashews, roughly
  chopped
few leaves of cilantro—
  optional

METHOD

Crack the eggs into a bowl and add the soy sauce and sesame oil, along with a grinding of black pepper. Beat together thoroughly.

Pour the peanut oil into a small (about 6-inch) nonstick frying pan over high heat. When the oil is hot, pour the beaten egg mixture into the pan and use a wooden or plastic spoon to move the egg around as it cooks, a little like making scrambled eggs. When there is more firm egg than loose, turn the heat down to medium.

Lay the shrimp on top of the omelet, followed by the bean sprouts. Fold the omelet in half over the filling and let everything warm through for 30 seconds.

Gently tip your omelet onto a plate and top with the red chile, cashew nuts and cilantro leaves, if using.

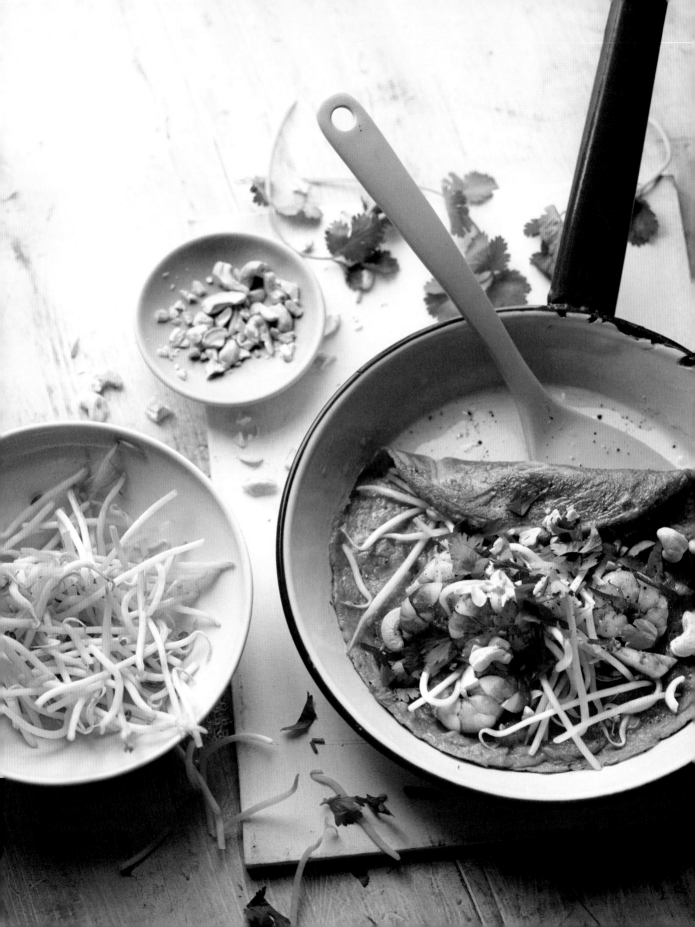

POACHED SALMON WITH BACON

Mmm, bacon and salmon. Yes, please! This dish is a real winner on flavor, and it's full of those essential omega-3 fatty acids that will help to keep you lean.

MAKE AHEAD
INGREDIENTS

2 skinless salmon fillets (about 8 oz each)
½ tbsp olive oil
2 slices Canadian bacon, sliced into ⅓-inch strips
1 zucchini, cut into half moons
7 oz midget trees (broccolini), any bigger stalks sliced in half lengthwise
8 cherry tomatoes
2 handfuls of baby spinach leaves
salt and pepper
¼ cup pine nuts
finely grated parmesan, to serve

METHOD

Bring a large saucepan of water to a boil. Carefully slide the salmon fillets into the water and reduce the heat to just simmering. Poach the fish for 10 minutes or until just cooked through. Using a slotted spoon, carefully lift the fish out of the water and drain well.

While the fish is cooking, heat the oil in a large frying pan over medium to high heat. When the oil is hot, fry the bacon for 1 minute, then add the zucchini and midget trees and fry for another minute. Throw in the cherry tomatoes and cook for another minute or until the tomatoes start to burst open and leak some of their delicious juices. Add the spinach and let it wilt down, then season with a little salt and a generous amount of pepper.

Divide the bacon and vegetable mixture between two plates, top with the poached salmon and finish with a scattering of pine nuts. Serve with a little finely grated parmesan.

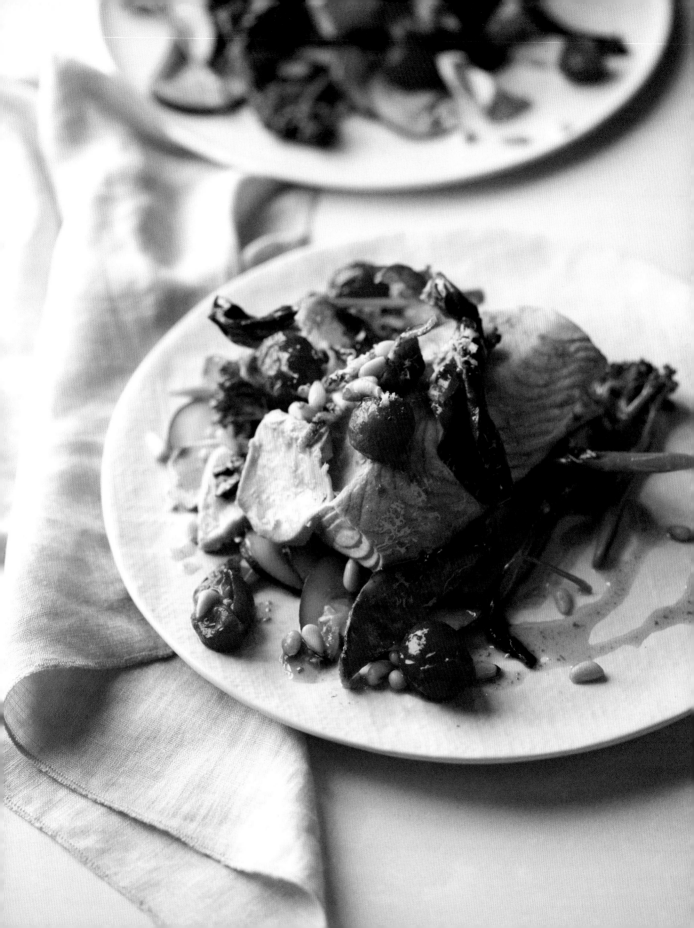

SEA BASS WITH SPICED CAULIFLOWER, PEAS AND PANEER

SERVES 2

The Indian fresh cheese known as paneer is very similar to halloumi, and it goes perfectly with the sea bass and cauliflower in this dish. Feel free to use halloumi if you can't find paneer. Garam masala is a pantry essential and brings a big boost of flavor to almost anything!

INGREDIENTS

1 small cauliflower, broken into florets
1 tbsp coconut oil
1 red onion, diced
¾ inch fresh ginger, finely chopped
5 oz paneer, roughly diced into ¾-inch cubes
1 tbsp garam masala
5 oz frozen peas
2 handfuls of baby spinach leaves
½ bunch of cilantro, leaves only, roughly chopped
4 sea bass fillets (4 oz each), skin on, but scaled
salt and pepper
juice of 1 lime

METHOD

Bring a large saucepan of water to a boil, then drop in the cauliflower florets and cook for 3 minutes. Drain in a sieve or colander, then rinse under cold running water. Leave the florets cooling in the sieve or colander.

In a large frying pan or wok, heat half the coconut oil over medium to high heat. Add the onion and stir-fry for 2 minutes or until just starting to soften, then add the ginger and stir-fry for another minute.

Add the paneer, garam masala and peas and keep stir-frying for 1–2 minutes, or until the peas have thawed and are warmed through. If the garam masala seems to be catching on the bottom of the pan and burning, just add a drizzle of water. Chuck in the spinach, cauliflower and cilantro and stir until the spinach has wilted.

In a separate frying pan, heat the rest of the coconut oil over medium to high heat. Season the fish fillets with salt and pepper and, when the oil is hot, lay the fish in the pan, skin side down. Fry without turning for 1–2 minutes until the skin is crisp, then flip the fish over and cook for a final minute.

Divide the paneer and vegetables between two plates and top with the sea bass. Finish with a squeeze of lime juice.

CODDLED EGGS WITH SPINACH AND BACON

Coddled eggs are basically steamed, creamy eggs. I love their texture, but if you would rather have poached or scrambled eggs, then go for it.

SERVES 1

INGREDIENTS

large knob of butter
2 large eggs
½ tbsp olive oil
4 slices Canadian bacon, sliced into ⅓-inch-wide thick strips
2 large handfuls of baby spinach leaves
salt and pepper
2 tbsp pine nuts

METHOD

Bring a large saucepan of water to a boil and set a steamer basket on top.

Drop a chunk of butter into two ramekins, then crack an egg into each one. When the water is boiling and there is a good amount of steam running through the steamer, carefully place the ramekins into the basket. Cover and steam the eggs for 6–10 minutes or until the whites are firm, but the yolks are still runny.

Meanwhile, heat the olive oil in a large frying pan over medium to high heat. Add the bacon and fry for 1–2 minutes or until crisp. Stir in the spinach and cook until it has wilted, then season with salt and pepper.

Serve up the coddled eggs with the bacon and spinach, topped with a sprinkling of pine nuts.

SERVES 2

SALMON WITH CAPERS AND CAPRESE SALAD

Close your eyes when you eat this and you could be in Italy: Caprese salad, capers and fresh basil. What a combo!

MAKE AHEAD

INGREDIENTS

¼ cup light olive oil
2 skinless salmon fillets
   (about 8 oz each)
1 tsp Dijon mustard
juice of ½ lemon
2 tsp capers
1 avocado, roughly diced
2 ripe tomatoes, roughly
   chopped
1 ball of mozzarella, torn
   into pieces
small handful of basil leaves
½ cup walnuts, roughly
   chopped

METHOD

Heat 1 tablespoon of the olive oil in a frying pan over medium to high heat. Add the salmon fillets and fry for 1–2 minutes on each side, by which time the fish should be lightly colored. Using a spatula, break the fish into large chunks and fry for another 2–3 minutes or until the fish is just cooked through. Remove the pan from the heat and transfer the salmon to a plate.

Mix together the mustard, lemon juice, capers and the remaining olive oil to make a dressing.

Arrange the avocado, tomatoes and mozzarella over two plates. Top with the salmon chunks, scatter with the basil leaves and walnuts, and finally spoon over the dressing.

★ **TOP TIP**

Buy herb plants, sit them in a window box or on a windowsill and you'll have free herbs forever.

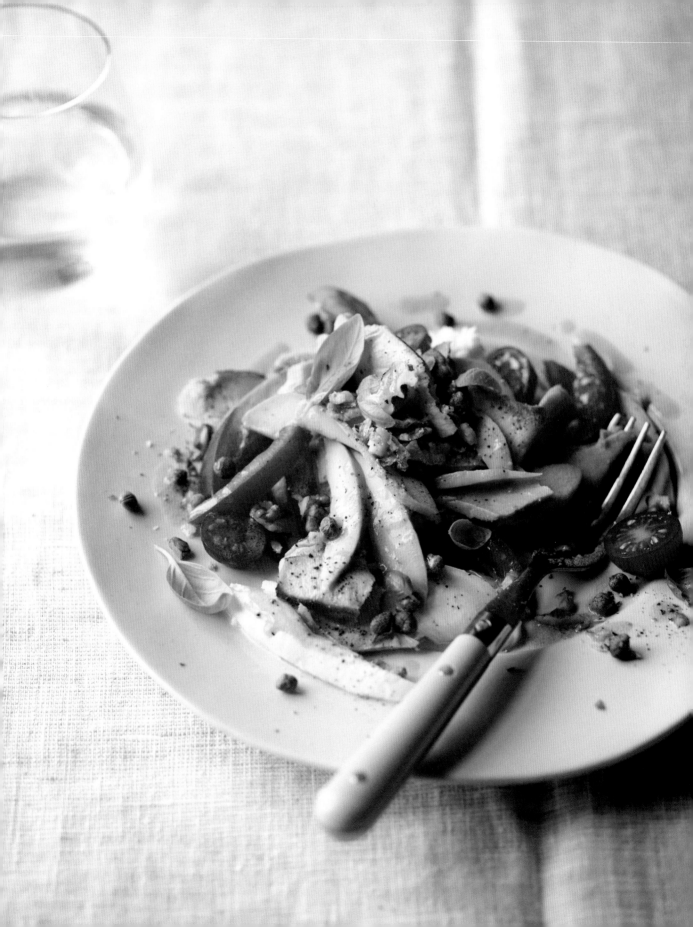

TERIYAKI SALMON WITH ZUCCHINI NOODLES

MAKE AHEAD

INGREDIENTS

½ tbsp coconut oil
8 oz skinless salmon fillet
2 scallions, finely sliced
¾ inch fresh ginger, finely
  chopped
2 tbsp light soy sauce
1 tbsp honey
½ tbsp rice wine vinegar
4 cherry tomatoes, cut in half
1 large zucchini, spiralized
  or sliced to make long
  noodle-like strands
2 tsp sesame oil

If you don't have a spiralizer, make the zucchini noodles by using a peeler to create long thin ribbons of zucchini, which you can then stack up and slice with a knife into noodle-like strips.

METHOD

Heat half of the coconut oil in a frying pan over medium to high heat. When the oil is melted and hot, slide in the salmon and fry for 2–3 minutes on each side or until lightly browned and almost cooked through.

Meanwhile, mix together the scallions, ginger, soy sauce, honey and vinegar to make a teriyaki sauce. Pour this into the pan with the salmon and let it bubble up, then remove the pan from the heat.

In another frying pan, heat the remaining coconut oil over high heat. Tumble in the tomatoes and stir-fry for 1 minute. Gently add the zucchini noodles and lightly toss for 1 minute just to warm through.

Plate up the noodles and tomatoes, then top with the teriyaki salmon. Finish with a little drizzle of sesame oil.

MAKE AHEAD
**(but reheat in the oven,
not in the microwave)**
GOOD TO FREEZE

INGREDIENTS

⅔ **cup rolled oats**
½ **cup ground almonds**
1 tbsp smoked paprika
salt and pepper
1 egg
**2 boneless, skinless chicken
   breasts (about 8 oz each)**
2 tbsp all-purpose flour
1 tbsp coconut oil
½ **cucumber, roughly
   chopped into ¾-inch pieces**
**1 large tomato, roughly
   chopped**
1 avocado, roughly chopped
1 tbsp olive oil
squeeze of lemon juice

MY OATY CHICKEN

Feeling stressed out after a long day at work? Cook this meal and you can take it out on your chicken, as you get to give it a good bash with a rolling pin or your fists to make it cook more quickly. Oh, and did I mention it's covered in an oaty, nutty crispy coating that tastes out of this world when you fry it in coconut oil?

METHOD

In a shallow dish, mix together the rolled oats, ground almonds, smoked paprika and a generous pinch of salt and pepper. Crack the egg into another shallow bowl and whisk.

Lay a large sheet of plastic wrap on your cutting board and place the chicken breasts on it, allowing room for them to spread, then place another sheet of plastic wrap on top. Using a rolling pin, meat hammer or other blunt instrument, bash the breasts until they are half their original thickness and flattened out. Remove the chicken breasts from the plastic wrap and dust all over with the flour, shaking them lightly to remove any excess, then dip into the beaten egg, again shaking off any excess. Finally, dunk the chicken breasts into the oat and almond mixture, pressing it on to cover both sides as well as you can.

Heat the coconut oil in a large nonstick frying pan over medium heat. Carefully lay the chicken breasts into the oil and fry for about 4 minutes on each side or until the chicken is cooked through. Check by cutting into the thickest part to make sure the meat is white, with no signs of pink. Transfer the chicken to paper towels to drain off any excess oil.

Mix together the cucumber, tomato, avocado, olive oil and lemon juice to make a quick salad, then serve alongside the oaty chicken.

MUSSELS IN COCONUT MILK

SERVES 2

If you've never tried mussels cooked in coconut milk, you're in for a treat. They make a nice change from fish or shrimp, and they taste great.

INGREDIENTS

1 tbsp coconut oil
2 star anise
6 scallions, finely sliced
2 cloves garlic, finely chopped
1 lemongrass stalk, bruised with the back of a knife
1 red chile, roughly chopped—remove the seeds if you don't like it hot
1 can (13.5 oz) full-fat coconut milk
4½ lb mussels, shells scrubbed and beards removed
2 tbsp fish sauce
small bunch of cilantro, leaves only, roughly chopped
2 limes

METHOD

Heat the coconut oil in a very large pan or wok for which you have a lid (or you can improvise with a large dinner plate or a sheet of foil). When the oil has melted, add the star anise, scallions, garlic, lemongrass and chile and stir-fry for 1 minute or until the scallions and garlic are starting to soften—by now the smell should be getting your appetite going too!

Pour in the coconut milk and bring to a boil, then reduce the heat and simmer for about 3 minutes to reduce the liquid a little. Check your mussels at this point: if there are any that are open and do not clamp shut when tapped, throw them away. Tumble the mussels into the coconut milk and give them a stir, then cover and cook for 3–4 minutes, shaking the pan every now and then. The mussels are cooked when their shells are fully open—be careful not to overcook, as that's how they become chewy. Discard any mussels that don't open up.

Remove the pan from the heat and stir in the fish sauce, half of the chopped cilantro and the juice of one of the limes. Divide the mussels between two bowls and garnish with the rest of the cilantro. Cut the other lime in half and serve on the side of the bowl, for squeezing.

★ Serve with a big portion of your favorite greens such as spinach, kale, broccoli, snow peas or green beans.

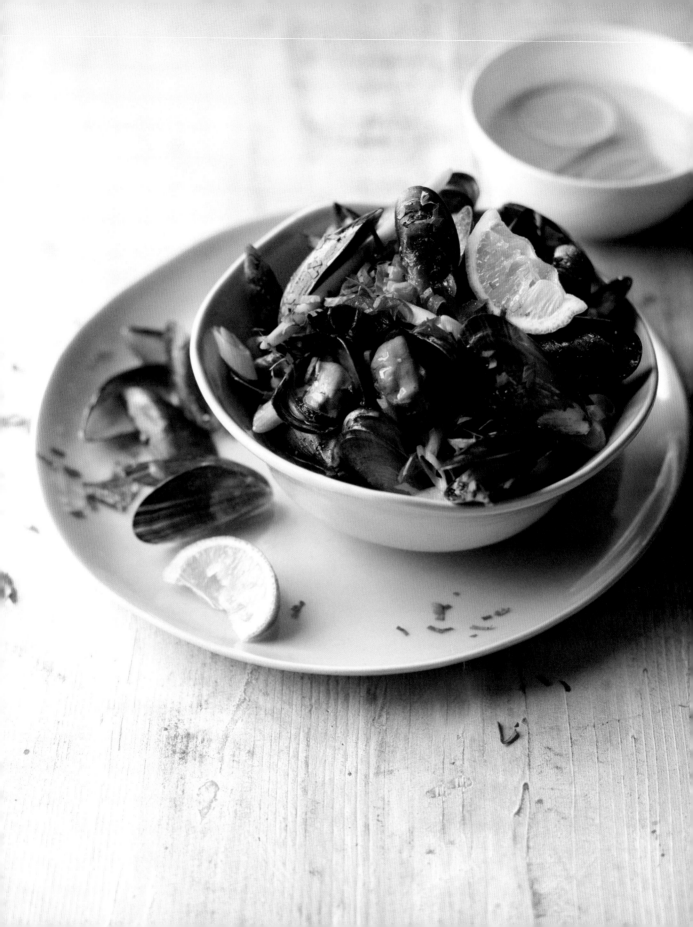

STEAK WITH SPICY CHORIZO, TOMATOES AND KALE

Ooh, steak and chorizo in one dish? Count me in! This is a real meat lover's dish. If you're not a fan of kale, you could always use spinach, but be sure to get your greens in.

INGREDIENTS

2 tbsp olive oil
2 (about 8 oz each) sirloin
  steaks, trimmed of
  visible fat
salt and pepper
3 oz Spanish (dry-cured)
  chorizo, diced
7 oz kale, thick stalks
  removed
8 cherry tomatoes, cut in half
1 tbsp sherry vinegar,
  or balsamic or red wine
  vinegar

METHOD

Bring a large saucepan of water to a boil, and place a frying pan over a high heat.

Rub the olive oil all over the steaks and season generously with salt and pepper. When the pan is very hot, carefully lay the steaks in it and fry for 2 minutes before flipping and frying for another 2 minutes. Transfer the steak to a plate and let rest.

Meanwhile, throw the chorizo into the same frying pan, turn the heat down to low and cook for about 2 minutes. At the same time, drop the kale into the boiling water and simmer for 1 minute, then drain in a sieve or colander.

Crank up the heat under the chorizo to maximum, then add the tomatoes to the pan and stir-fry for 1 minute. Pour in the vinegar and let it bubble away to almost nothing. Add the kale and toss to combine everything thoroughly.

Remove from the heat and season to taste with salt and pepper. Place a steak on each plate and top with the delicious stir-fry.

CLASSIC SMOKED SALMON AND SCRAMBLED EGGS

SERVES 2

The king of healthy breakfasts is a true Lean in 15 dish!
If you're always in a rush in the morning, this one's for you.
Scrambling the eggs on a low heat with butter gives them
a seriously creamy texture.

INGREDIENTS

6 eggs
4 tsp butter, roughly chopped
pepper
6 slices smoked salmon,
  cut into ⅓-inch-thick strips
small bunch of chives,
  finely sliced
handful of baby spinach
  leaves, to serve

METHOD

Bring a saucepan of water to a boil.

Crack the eggs into a large heatproof bowl and add the
butter, along with a good grinding of pepper. Whisk the eggs
together, then sit the bowl over the pan of boiling water and
immediately reduce the heat to a simmer. Cook the eggs
for about 10 minutes, stirring regularly. As the eggs begin to
scramble, add the smoked salmon and the chives, and keep
cooking the eggs until they reach your preferred consistency—
the longer you cook them, the firmer they'll get.

Serve up these luxurious eggs with a big handful of spinach
and a final grinding of black pepper.

SEA BASS WITH BRAZIL NUTS, KALE AND POMEGRANATE

Sea bass with nuts and pomegranate—such a great combination of flavors and packed with goodness. This is a dish to impress your friends at a dinner party!

SERVES 1

MAKE AHEAD
INGREDIENTS

2 tbsp olive oil
2 skin-on sea bass fillets
  (about 4 oz each)
salt and pepper
3 oz kale, thick stalks removed
4 midget trees (broccolini),
  any bigger stalks sliced in
  half lengthwise
2 tbsp pomegranate seeds
1 oz Brazil nuts, chopped
1 red chile, finely sliced—
  remove the seeds if you
  don't like it hot

METHOD

Bring a saucepan of water to a boil.

Meanwhile, heat half of the olive oil in a frying pan over medium to high heat. Season the sea bass with salt and pepper and, when the oil is hot, carefully lay the fish in the pan, skin side down. Cook, without turning, for 2–3 minutes, then carefully flip it over. Remove the pan from the heat and let the fish finish cooking in the residual heat.

Drop the kale and midget trees into the boiling water and simmer for 2 minutes. Drain in a sieve or colander, then rinse under cold running water. Transfer the vegetables to a bowl and add the rest of the olive oil, along with the pomegranate seeds, Brazil nuts and chile. Gently toss everything together.

Pile the vegetables onto the plate, sit the fish on top, and tuck in.

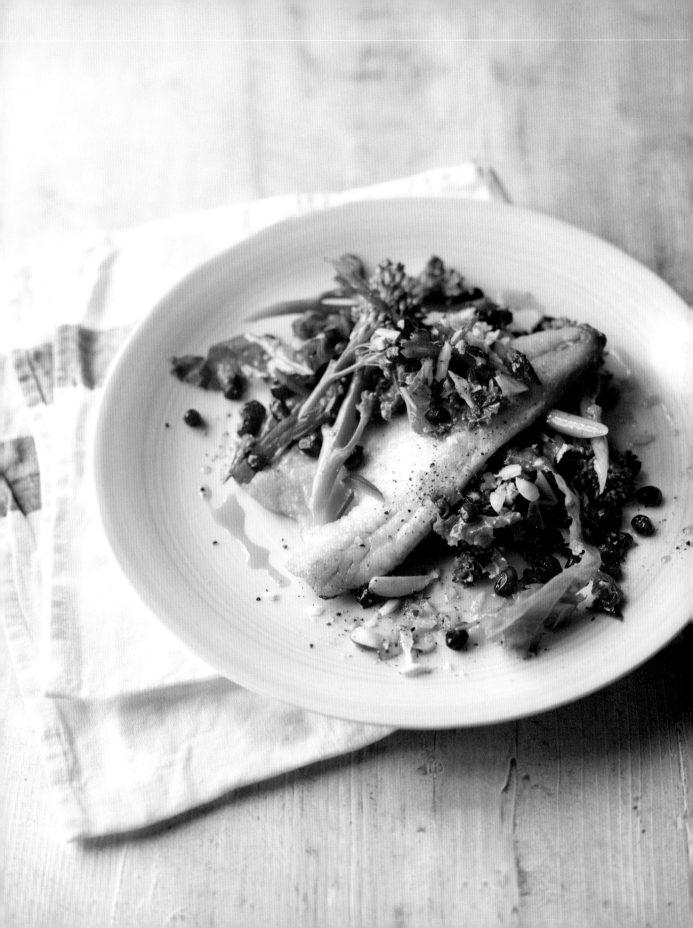

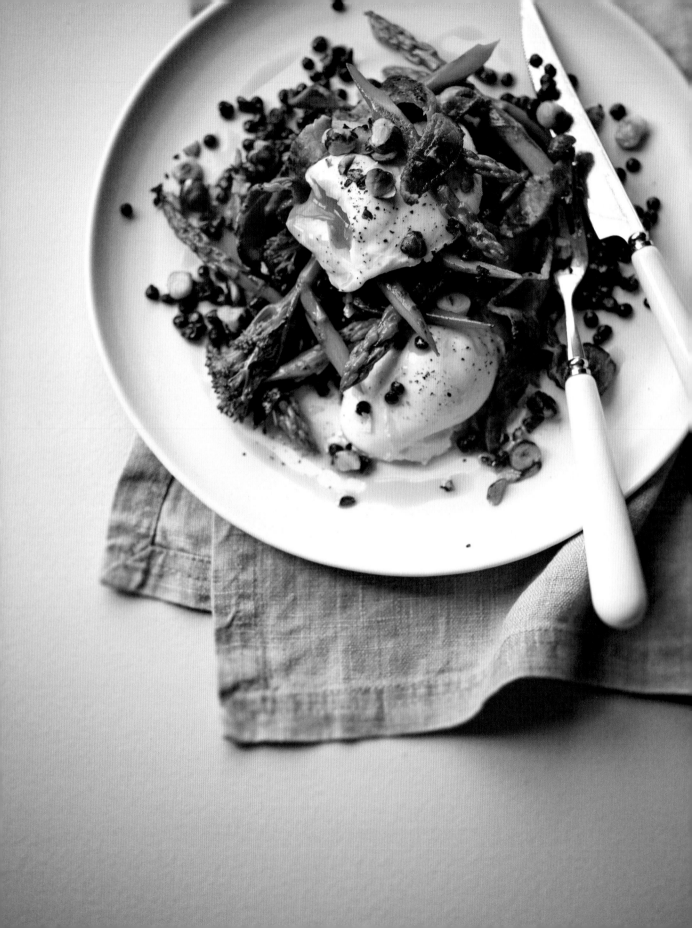

GRIDDLED MIDGET TREES AND SPEARS WITH EGGS

SERVES 2

What can I say? You know how obsessed I am with midget trees! Well, here's a breakfast idea I'm sure you'll love as much as I do.

INGREDIENTS

8 spears of asparagus, woody parts of stalks removed
8 midget trees (broccolini)
2 slices Canadian bacon
salt and pepper
5 oz pre-cooked Puy lentils
4 eggs
glug of olive oil
splash of sherry vinegar
2 tbsp toasted and chopped hazelnuts

METHOD

Bring a large saucepan of water to a boil and place a griddle pan over high heat. It's probably best to throw open a window too, as griddling always seems to set the smoke alarm off . . .

When the griddle pan is hot, place the spears, trees and bacon directly onto it, sprinkling the vegetables with a little salt and pepper. Cook for 3–4 minutes, turning regularly—you're after crispy bacon and lightly chargrilled vegetables.

Heat the lentils in the microwave according to the package instructions.

Carefully crack your eggs into the hot water, reducing the heat until the water is just "burping." Cook the eggs for about 4 minutes for a runny yolk, then carefully lift them out with a slotted spoon and drain on paper towels.

Once the veg are all cooked, scoop them up and drop them into a large bowl. Remove the bacon and roughly chop, then add to the bowl too, along with the olive oil, sherry vinegar and lentils. Season to taste with salt and pepper and toss the whole lot together before piling onto plates. Top with the poached eggs and finish with the toasted hazelnuts.

DUCK, GREEN BEANS AND WALNUTS

MAKE AHEAD
INGREDIENTS

1 tbsp olive oil
8 oz boneless, skinless
  duck breast, sliced into
  ¾-inch-thick strips
salt and pepper
4 oz green beans
1 tbsp walnut oil
6 tbsp walnuts
2 tbsp sun-dried tomatoes

Oh, hello, healthy fats! Although this feels like a high-end bistro dish, it's ready in minutes. And as it's just as tasty eaten at room temperature, it works very well as a packed lunch too.

METHOD

Bring a large saucepan of water to a boil.

Heat the olive oil in a frying pan over medium to high heat. Season the duck breast with salt and pepper. When the oil is hot, add the duck and fry, stirring occasionally, for about 3 minutes or until the duck is cooked through and lightly golden in places.

Meanwhile, drop the beans into the boiling water and simmer for 1 minute. Drain in a sieve or colander, then rinse under cold running water. Tip the beans into a bowl and add the walnut oil, walnuts and sun-dried tomatoes. Season generously with salt and pepper, then toss everything together.

Arrange the green beans and walnuts on a plate and top with the duck.

MAKE AHEAD
GOOD TO FREEZE
INGREDIENTS

½ tbsp coconut oil
½ red onion, diced
1 red or yellow bell pepper,
   thinly sliced
½ zucchini, diced
10 oz ready-made turkey
   meatballs (available at
   most supermarkets)
1 can (14 oz) chopped
   tomatoes
¾ oz feta, crumbled
½ bunch of parsley, leaves
   only, roughly chopped—
   optional

TURKEY MEATBALLS WITH FETA

These meatballs were a hit on Instagram, ranking as one of my most popular videos. The cheesy sauce also tastes great with beef meatballs. Feel free to throw in any extra veg you have left in the fridge too.

METHOD

Heat the coconut oil in a large frying pan over medium to high heat. Add the onion, bell pepper and zucchini, and stir-fry for 2 minutes until the vegetables begin to soften and wilt.

Increase the heat to maximum and roll the meatballs into the pan. Fry for 2–3 minutes, moving them frequently so they brown all over.

Pour in the chopped tomatoes and bring to a boil, then reduce the heat and simmer for 5 minutes, or until the meatballs are fully cooked through. To check, cut the largest one in half and make sure all the meat has turned from pink to white.

Remove the pan from the heat, crumble over the feta and sprinkle with parsley, if using.

★ TOP TIP

If you can't find ready-made turkey meatballs in your supermarket, simply buy ground turkey and season it with a generous amount of salt and pepper. Create some extra flavor by adding in a pinch of dried oregano, parsley or Cajun spice. Knead for a minute and then form into golfball-sized meatballs.

SERVES 2

LAMB KOFTAS WITH GREEK SALAD

This is a great summer dish and is brilliant on the grill. The fresh crispness of the salad cuts through the richness of the meat. If you want to change it up, ground beef works well with this recipe too.

MAKE AHEAD
GOOD TO FREEZE
(the koftas, not the salad!)
INGREDIENTS

¾ lb lean ground lamb
2 tsp ground cinnamon
2 tsp ground cumin
4 scallions, finely sliced
2 cloves garlic, finely chopped
salt and pepper
½ cucumber, roughly
  chopped into big chunks
1 large tomato, roughly
  chopped into big chunks
16 black olives
splash of sherry vinegar
small handful of mint leaves,
  to serve—optional

METHOD

Preheat the broiler to high.

Tip the lamb into a bowl. Add the cinnamon and cumin, scallions, garlic and a generous pinch of salt and pepper, then mix the whole lot together thoroughly—I find the best way is to dig your hands in there.

Mold the mixture into 4 equal-sized sausage shapes around a skewer and place on a broiler pan or a baking sheet. Broil the koftas for 5 minutes on each side or until well browned and cooked through.

Meanwhile, toss the cucumber, tomato, olives and vinegar together in a bowl.

Serve your koftas with this chunky salad—and an artistic scattering of mint leaves, if you like.

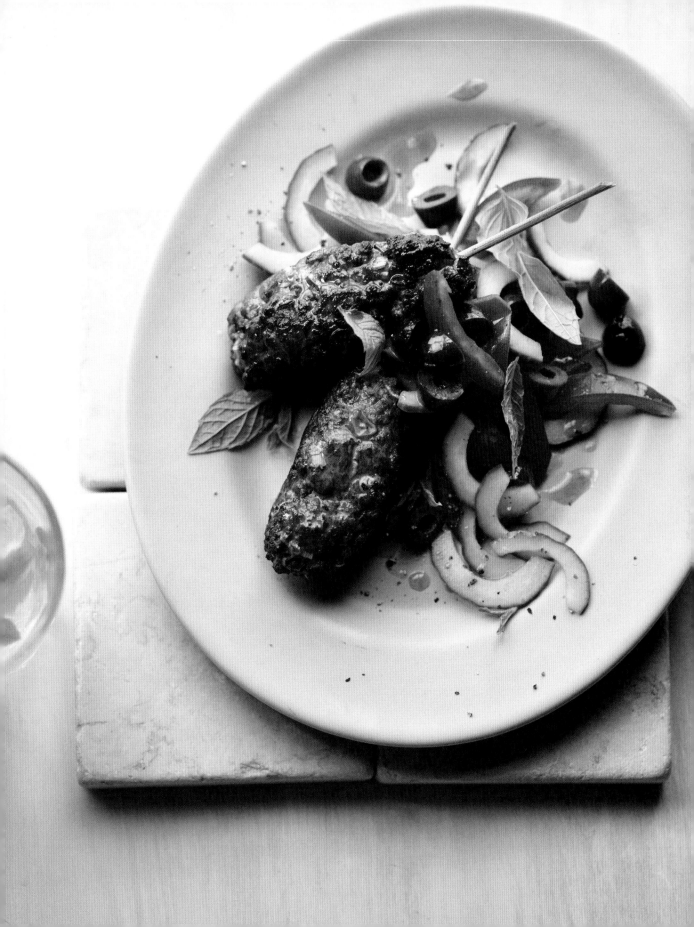

COCONUT AND CASHEW DAAL

LONGER RECIPE
MAKE AHEAD
GOOD TO FREEZE
INGREDIENTS

9 oz yellow split peas
(available in most
supermarkets)
1 tbsp coconut oil
1 small red onion, roughly
diced
1 tsp cumin seeds
1 cinnamon stick, broken
in two
1 fresh bay leaf, or 2 dried
4 cloves garlic, finely chopped
2 inches fresh ginger, finely
chopped
1 green chile, split lengthwise
1 tbsp garam masala
1 tsp ground turmeric
1 can (14 oz) full-fat coconut
milk
2 cups warm vegetable stock
7 oz cashews
2 large handfuls of baby
spinach leaves
bunch of cilantro, leaves
only, roughly chopped

A lovely vegetarian option to try. This is going to take rather longer than most of my recipes (about an hour for this one), but it's time well spent, as it tastes amazing.

METHOD

Place the split peas in a large bowl and cover with warm water from the tap. Leave to soak while you cook the onion and spices.

Melt the coconut oil in a large saucepan over medium heat. Add the onion and cook for 3–4 minutes until just soft. Add the cumin seeds, cinnamon and bay leaves and stir-fry for 45 seconds, then add the garlic, ginger and chile and cook for 1 minute. Sprinkle in the garam masala and turmeric and stir-fry for 30 seconds.

Drain the split peas and add to the pan, along with the coconut milk and half of the vegetable stock. Bring to a boil and simmer for about 30 minutes or until the split peas are completely tender.

Meanwhile, pour the rest of the vegetable stock over the cashews and leave to soak for 10 minutes. Tip the nuts and stock into a blender and blend until smooth.

When the split peas are tender, add the cashew cream and the spinach, then stir until the spinach has wilted into the daal. Remove from the heat and stir in the cilantro before gobbling down your yummy daal.

★ Serve with a big portion of your favorite greens such as spinach, kale, broccoli, snow peas or green beans.

LONGER RECIPE
MAKE AHEAD
GOOD TO FREEZE
INGREDIENTS

3 eggplants, cut lengthwise
  into slices about ¼ inch
  thick
about ½ cup olive oil
salt and pepper
1 large red onion, diced
3 cloves garlic, finely chopped
2¼ lb ground turkey
1 tsp ground cinnamon
1 tbsp tomato paste
1¼ cups chicken stock
2 tsp dried oregano
1 ball of mozzarella
  (about 8 oz)
¼ cup finely grated parmesan
bunch of parsley, leaves
  only, roughly chopped

TURKEY MOUSSAKA

Broiled eggplant is hard to beat—and in this moussaka, it becomes perfect dinner-party fodder. Even better, it can all be done in advance, so it's fuss-free. This dish actually takes more like 1 hour and 15 minutes to make, but for much of that time it looks after itself in the oven.

METHOD

Preheat the broiler to high. Lay a single layer of eggplant slices on a broiler pan or a baking sheet, drizzle with a little olive oil and season with salt and pepper. Slide under the broiler and cook for 2 minutes on each side. When cooked (soft to the touch and looking a little shriveled), transfer the eggplant slices to a plate and repeat the process until they are all cooked and sitting happily on the plate.

Heat a splash of olive oil in a large saucepan over medium to high heat. Add the onion and garlic and stir-fry for 3–4 minutes until beginning to soften. Increase the heat to high and add the turkey, cinnamon, tomato paste, chicken stock and oregano. Bring the whole lot up to a boil and leave to simmer for 20 minutes.

Preheat the oven to 375°F.

Pour about a quarter of the turkey mixture into a deep baking dish. Tear up half a ball of mozzarella and scatter over the turkey mixture, then lay a third of the broiled eggplant slices on top (it doesn't matter if they overlap slightly). Repeat the process until you have 3 layers of turkey mixture and 3 layers of eggplant, then finish with the final quarter of the turkey.

Scatter the parmesan over the top and cook the moussaka in the oven for about 30 minutes until heated through and golden brown. To finish your dish, sprinkle over the fresh parsley.

LONGER RECIPE
MAKE AHEAD
GOOD TO FREEZE
INGREDIENTS

2 large knobs of butter
1 large leek, washed and
   chopped into ¾-inch pieces
7 oz mushrooms, roughly
   chopped
1¼ lb boneless, skinless
   chicken breast, cut into
   bite-sized pieces
1 cup chicken stock
1 tbsp cornstarch
½ cup heavy cream
2 large handfuls of baby
   spinach leaves
about 6 sheets of phyllo
   pastry
drizzle of olive oil
salad or veg, to serve

JOE'S CHICKEN PIE

If you love chicken pie, this recipe won't disappoint. It's actually Lean in about 60 minutes, but is such a nice treat that you won't mind the extra effort. Plus, there's cream and butter in it, so you know it's going to taste incredible.

METHOD

Preheat the oven to 375°F.

Heat the butter in a large frying pan over medium to high heat. Add the leek and mushrooms and fry for 2–3 minutes until they just start to soften. Crank up the heat to high, add the chicken pieces and fry for another 2 minutes—the chicken won't be cooked through at this point—then pour in the chicken stock and let it come to a simmer.

Meanwhile, mix the cornstarch with 2 tablespoons of water until smooth, then pour into the pan, along with the cream. Bring back to a boil, stirring gently, and cook until the sauce thickens. Remove from the heat and stir in the spinach, then tip the whole lot into an oval baking dish about 11 × 6 inches. Set aside to cool a little.

Take a sheet of phyllo and roughly crumple it in your hands—there is no right or wrong to this method! Place the crumpled phyllo on top of the chicken filling in the dish and repeat with the remaining phyllo sheets.

Drizzle the pastry with olive oil, then bake the pie for about 20 minutes, by which time the phyllo will have crisped up and turned golden brown in places.

Serve up your pie with fresh salad or some vegetables.

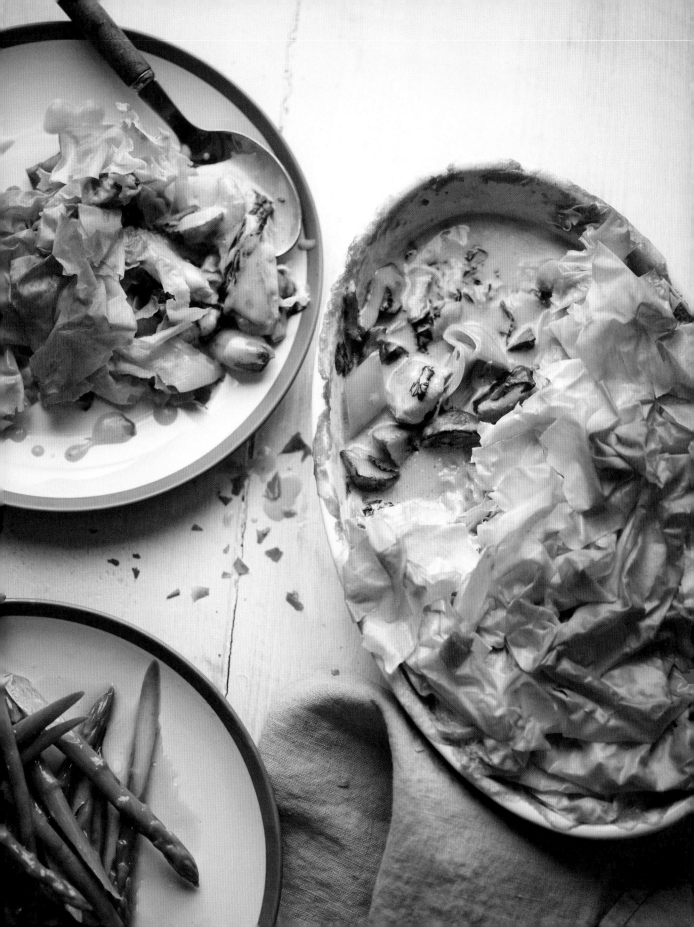

POST-WORKOUT CARBOHYDRATE-REFUEL RECIPES

4

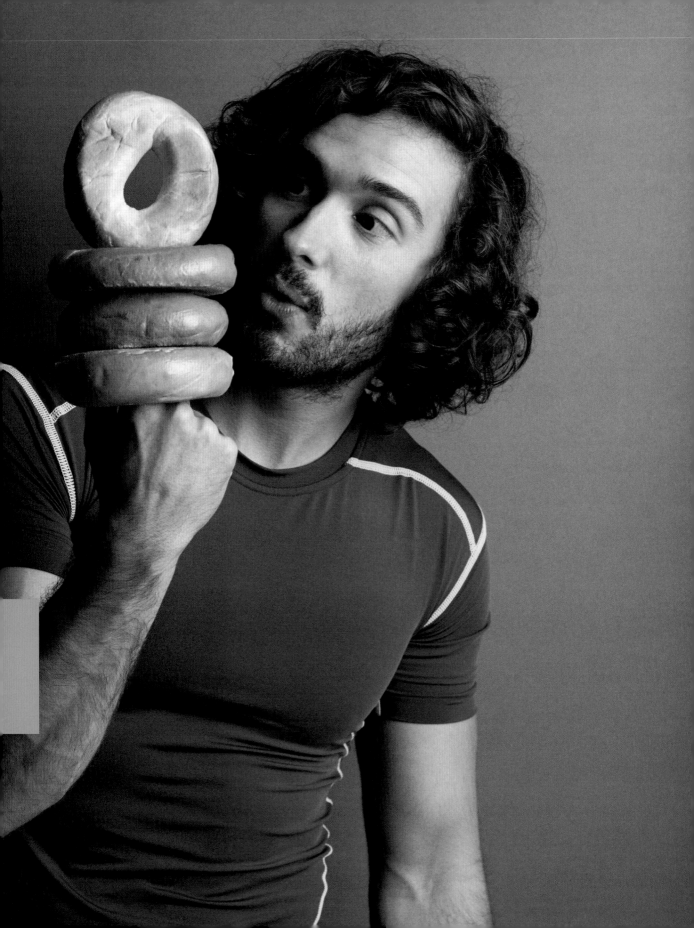

BANANA AND BLUEBERRY OVERNIGHT OATS

SERVES 1

This is a quick and easy breakfast to have ready to go, after jump-starting your day with a morning workout.

INGREDIENTS

1 banana, roughly chopped
⅓ cup full-fat yogurt
1 cup almond milk
1 scoop (30g) strawberry
protein powder
1¼ cups rolled oats
handful of pistachios or
other nuts, blueberries and
raspberries to serve

METHOD

Place the banana, yogurt, almond milk and protein powder into a blender and blend until smooth. Pour the mixture into a bowl and stir in the oats, then cover and refrigerate for at least 4 hours, preferably overnight.

When ready to eat, top with the nuts, blueberries and raspberries.

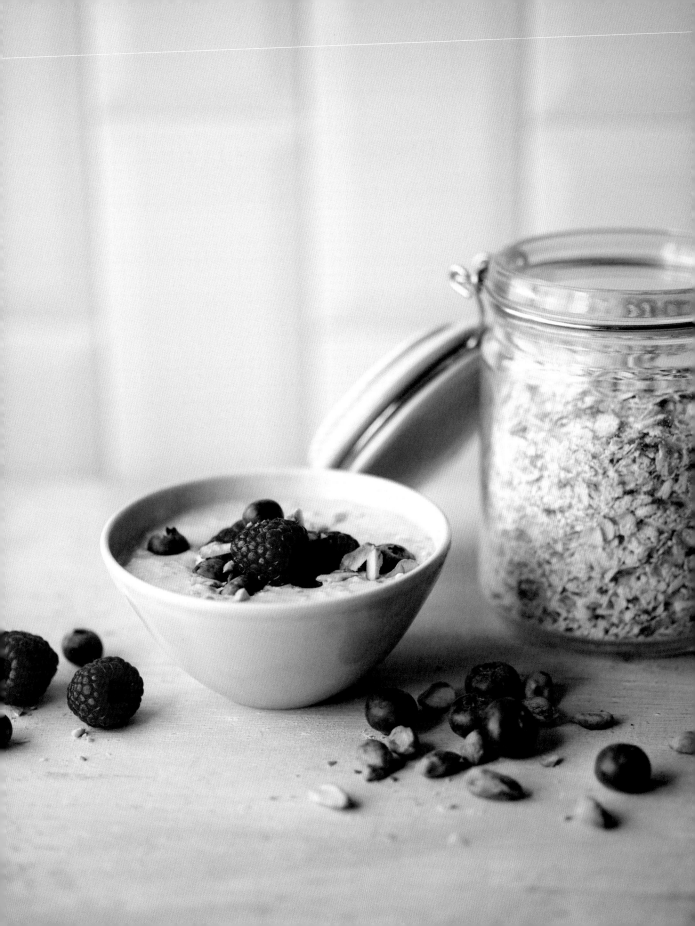

BIG McLEAN MUFFIN

**SERVES
1**

The thought of one of these waiting for you once you've finished your workout is enough to get you through those last reps. For the best poached eggs, use the freshest eggs possible.

INGREDIENTS

2 eggs

2 tsp coconut oil

5 cherry tomatoes

2 massive handfuls of baby spinach leaves

1 large English muffin

1 lb sliced deli-style ham or smoked ham, trimmed of visible fat

1 red chile, finely sliced—optional

METHOD

Bring a saucepan of water to a boil. Carefully crack your eggs into the hot water, reducing the heat until the water is just "burping." Cook the eggs for about 4 minutes for runny yolks, then carefully lift them out with a slotted spoon and drain on paper towels.

Meanwhile, heat the coconut oil in a large frying pan over medium to high heat. Add the tomatoes and toss in the hot oil for 1–2 minutes or until they are lightly browned and blistered. At this point, throw in the spinach and toss with the tomatoes until wilted, then remove the pan from the heat.

Toast your muffin, top with the ham and spoon over the tomatoes and spinach, then finish with the poached eggs and some sliced red chile, if using.

WINNER'S PROTEIN PANCAKES

Oooh, I can eat pancakes and get lean? Yes please—sold! These may look naughty, but they're actually the perfect post-workout treat, so stack 'em up and enjoy. You've earned them!

INGREDIENTS

1 banana, roughly chopped
1 scoop (30g) vanilla protein
   powder
1 egg
⅓ cup rolled oats
1 tbsp coconut oil
full-fat Greek yogurt,
   blueberries and raspberries,
   to serve

METHOD

Whizz up the banana, protein powder, egg and oats in a blender to make your batter.

Heat up half the coconut oil in a nonstick frying pan over medium heat. Pour little puddles of batter into the pan— I usually get 3 pancakes, with about half the batter in the pan at once. Cook for about 1 minute on each side. Remove and repeat the process with the rest of the batter.

Serve with a dollop of yogurt and a few berries (see picture pg. 107).

SERVES 1

INGREDIENTS

scant 1 cup rolled oats
large handful of blueberries
handful of ice cubes
1 banana, roughly chopped
1 scoop (30g) vanilla or
    strawberry protein powder
1 tbsp chia seeds
1 cup coconut water or water

BLUEBERRY AND BANANA PROTEIN SHAKE

This is a great way to get a load of vitamins into your diet, as it's so easy to make and transport (you can have it on your morning commute). I really recommend a good blender: they're worth their weight in gold. Just remember that protein shakes are fine to have now and then, but they aren't meant to replace actual food—so keep mixing it up!

METHOD

Place all the ingredients in a blender and blend until smooth.

★ TOP TIP

Chia seeds were an important food for the Aztecs and Mayans back in the day. They prized them for their ability to provide sustainable energy—in fact, "chia" is the ancient Mayan word for "strength." Don't be fooled by their size! As a good source of fiber, protein and antioxidants, these little seeds pack a nutritional power punch.

SERVES 1

INGREDIENTS

generous ¾ cup almond milk
1 granny smith apple, cored
    and roughly chopped
2 large handfuls (4 oz) of
    baby spinach leaves
1 scoop (30g) vanilla protein
    powder
scant 1 cup rolled oats

INCREDIBLE HULK SMOOTHIE

This is green and good for you. I like to leave the skin on my apple, as it is full of nutrients, but you may prefer not to—either way is fine! Enjoy.

METHOD

Place all the ingredients in a blender with a handful of ice and blitz until smooth.

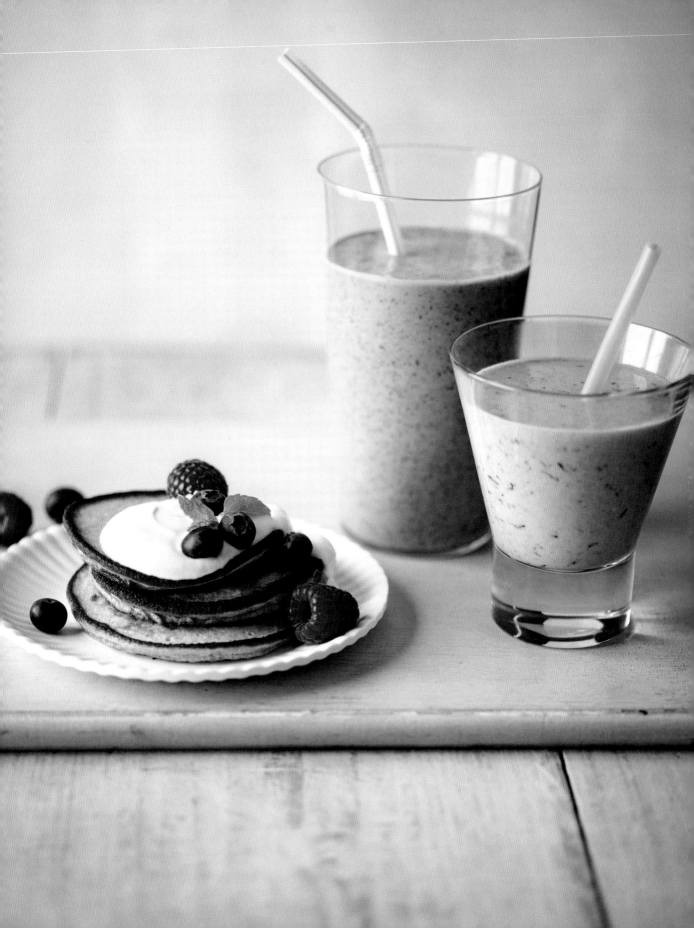

BUILD-UP BAGEL

Long live the build-up bagel. For some reason, people on my plan go absolutely bonkers for this post-workout bagel. I think they feel naughty eating it—but, like I say, you've just trained and earned those carbs, so no need to feel guilty. Go for good-quality cooked meat, not the nasty cheap re-formed stuff. If you don't want to bother with poaching the egg, you could always just boil and slice it instead.

**SERVES
1**

INGREDIENTS

1 egg
1 plain bagel
2 tsp chipotle paste or
  barbecue sauce
1 tbsp full-fat Greek yogurt
large handful of arugula
1 tomato, sliced
5 oz deli-style cooked turkey
  or chicken breast
2½ oz deli-style sliced
  roast beef

METHOD

Bring a saucepan of water to a boil. Carefully crack your egg into the hot water, reducing the heat until the water is just "burping." Cook the egg for about 4 minutes for a runny yolk, then carefully lift it out with a slotted spoon and drain on paper towels.

Slice the bagel in half and toast it for a couple of minutes.

Spread the toasted bagel evenly with the chipotle paste or barbecue sauce and the yogurt, and then begin building your bagel: start with the arugula and tomato, followed by the turkey or chicken and the beef, then the poached egg. Finally, stick the top on the bagel and get munching!

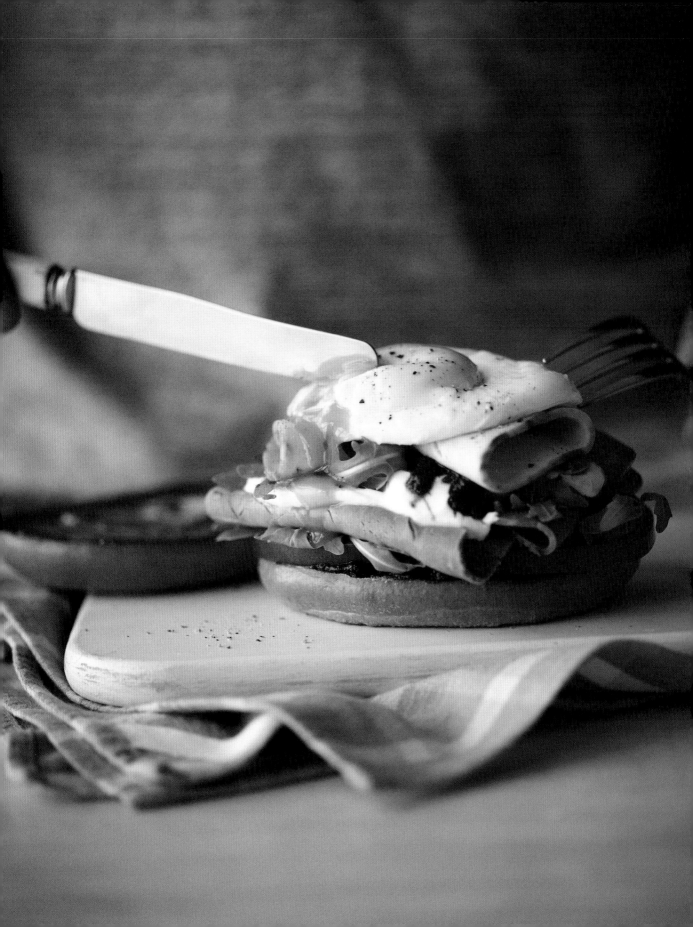

CHICKEN AND NEW POTATO HASH

SERVES 1

Standing around waiting for potatoes to boil? No, thanks. Throw them into the microwave instead and cook them in half the time. This is proper comfort food—a real reward after a workout. You won't feel hungry after this one.

INGREDIENTS

7 oz new potatoes
½ tbsp coconut oil
7 oz boneless, skinless chicken breast, sliced into ⅓-inch-thick strips
4 scallions, sliced
3 oz snow peas
1 egg
1 tsp smoked paprika
2 large handfuls of baby spinach leaves
pinch of red pepper flakes, if you like it hot

METHOD

Prick the new potatoes with a fork and blast them in the microwave for 8 minutes.

Meanwhile, melt the oil in a large frying pan over medium to high heat. Add the chicken and fry for 2 minutes, stirring occasionally—you want the chicken to be browned in places. Add the scallions and the snow peas and stir-fry for 1 minute, then remove from the heat. You should now have about 4 minutes until your spuds ping, so time for a quick set of push-ups—go!

Bring a saucepan of water to a boil. Carefully crack your egg into the hot water, reducing the heat until the water is just "burping." Cook the egg for about 4 minutes for a runny yolk, then carefully lift it out with a slotted spoon and drain on paper towels.

Once the spuds have pinged, carefully (maybe using a knife and fork, as they'll be very hot) halve them, cutting any larger ones into quarters. Return the frying pan to high heat, then slide in the potatoes and fry, without turning, for 3–4 minutes or until the potatoes are beginning to brown in places. Add the smoked paprika and spinach, then toss to coat all the ingredients evenly and wilt the spinach.

Spoon up your hash, top with the poached egg and finish with a little pepper flake fire, if you want.

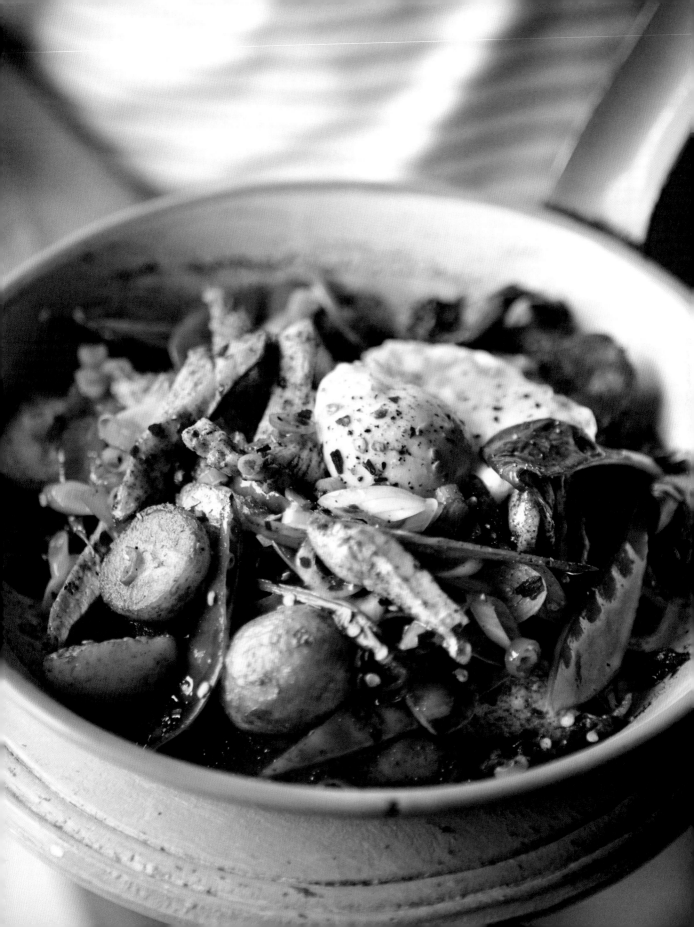

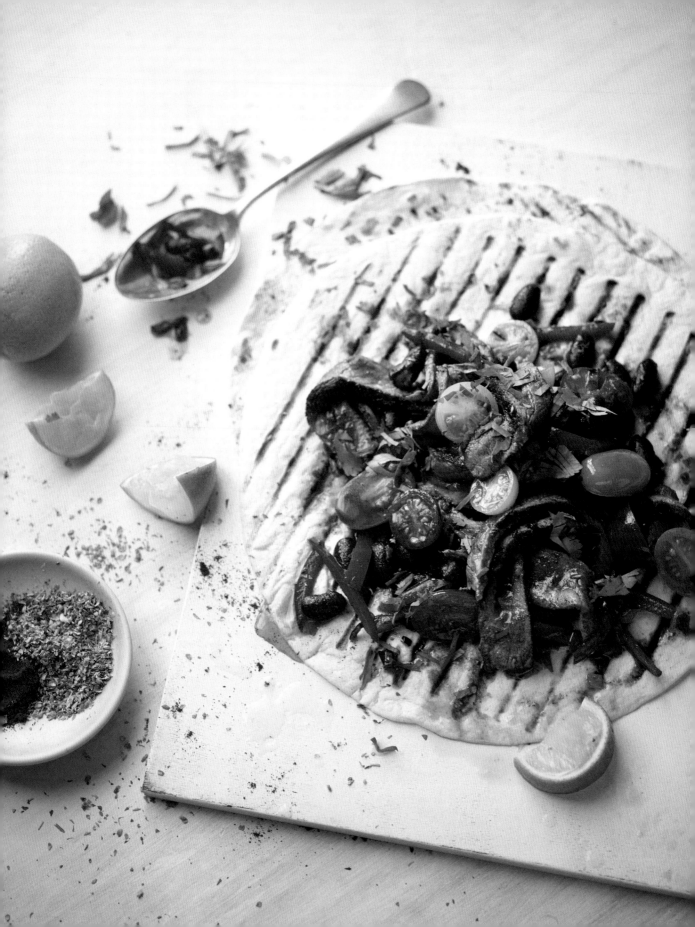

BAD-BOY BURRITO

You've just worked out and earned your carbs. This monster burrito needs two hands to eat, and is a proper treat that's guaranteed to fill you up and leave you feeling like a hero. It's also really quick and easy to make up and then carry with you to work. For a change, try using chicken instead of beef, or pita bread instead of tortillas.

MAKE AHEAD

INGREDIENTS

- 1 tbsp coconut oil
- 1 lb sirloin steak, trimmed of visible fat and cut into ⅓-inch-thick slices
- 1 red onion, roughly chopped
- 1 red bell pepper, roughly sliced
- 1 clove garlic, finely chopped
- 1 tsp paprika
- 1 tsp dried oregano
- 6 cherry tomatoes, roughly chopped
- salt and pepper
- 1 can (15 oz) kidney beans, drained and rinsed
- 2 large tortilla wraps
- small bunch of cilantro, leaves only, roughly chopped
- squeeze of lime juice

METHOD

Heat the coconut oil in a large frying pan over high heat. Add the steak and fry for 1–2 minutes, turning the meat a couple of times. Throw in the onion, bell pepper and garlic and stir-fry for a minute or two. Add the paprika, oregano and tomatoes, season with salt and pepper, and toss everything together for a minute. Chuck in the kidney beans and cook for another minute, by which time the beans should be warmed through.

Pile half the mixture along the middle of each wrap, then top with some chopped cilantro and finish with a squeeze of lime juice. Roll up and gobble down.

MAKE AHEAD
(the chili not the sweet
potato)

INGREDIENTS

1 sweet potato
2 tsp coconut oil
3 scallions, finely sliced
8 oz 95% lean ground beef
1 tsp ground cumin
1 tsp smoked paprika
2 tsp tomato paste
1 cup canned kidney beans,
  drained and rinsed
½ cup beef stock
1 tbsp full-fat Greek yogurt

SWEET POTATO WITH CHILI

Sweet potato is one of my favorite carb sources and when you combine it with a quick beef chili, it's a real banger. To make this Lean in 15, I use a microwave to cook the potato, but if you'd rather boil the sweet potato or bake it in the oven, go for it.

METHOD

Prick the sweet potato a couple of times with a fork, then blast it in the microwave for 5 minutes. Leave it to rest for 30 seconds and then blast it for a further 3–4 minutes. Set aside, loosely covered in foil, until needed.

Meanwhile, melt the coconut oil in a large frying pan over high heat. Stir in the scallions and beef and stir-fry for about 4 minutes, breaking up any chunks of meat as you go. When the meat is browned, sprinkle in the cumin and paprika and cook for 30 seconds before adding the tomato paste. Stir-fry for another 30 seconds, then add the kidney beans and beef stock. Bring to a simmer and cook for 1 minute.

Split open the sweet potato and serve with the quick chili— and some cooling yogurt.

★ Serve with a big portion of your favorite greens such as spinach, kale, broccoli, snow peas or green beans.

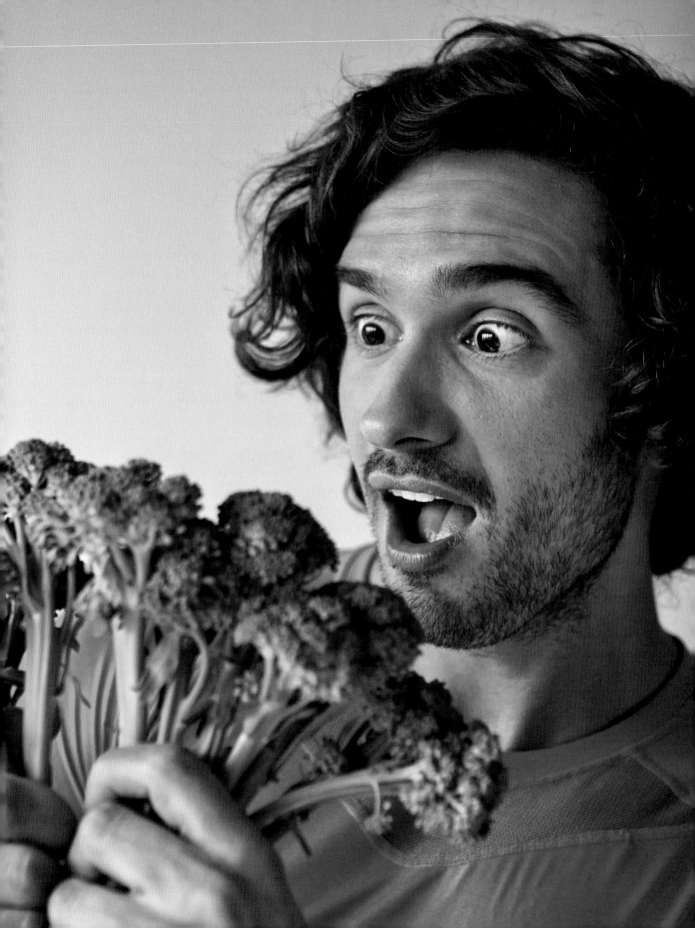

SHRIMP AND NOODLE STIR-FRY

SERVES 1

This is about as lean as they come. One wok, no hassle and another chance to throw some midget trees around. This makes a great lunch, too, so cook double and take the extra in a lunch box to work the next day.

MAKE AHEAD

INGREDIENTS

½ tbsp coconut oil
3 scallions, finely sliced
1 clove garlic, finely chopped
½ lb raw shrimp, peeled
2 oz snow peas, sliced in half
3 baby corn, sliced in half
4 midget trees (broccolini),
  any bigger stalks sliced
  in half lengthwise
7 oz refrigerated stir-fry
  noodles
2 tbsp light soy sauce
1 tbsp fish sauce

METHOD

Melt the coconut oil in a wok or large frying pan over medium to high heat. Add the scallions and garlic and stir-fry for 1 minute. Add the shrimp and continue to stir for a further minute.

Toss in the snow peas, corn and midget trees, along with about 2 tablespoons of water. Let the water bubble up and create steam to cook the vegetables. Add the noodles, breaking up the clumps with your fingers as you drop them in. Toss to mix the noodles with the other ingredients, then stir-fry for a minute until the noodles are warmed through and soft.

Remove from the heat, pour in the soy sauce and fish sauce, then give the whole lot one last stir before piling onto a plate and munching away.

★ TOP TIP

For a gluten-free meal, swap the soy sauce for tamari, and use rice noodles instead of the refrigerated stiry-fry noodles.

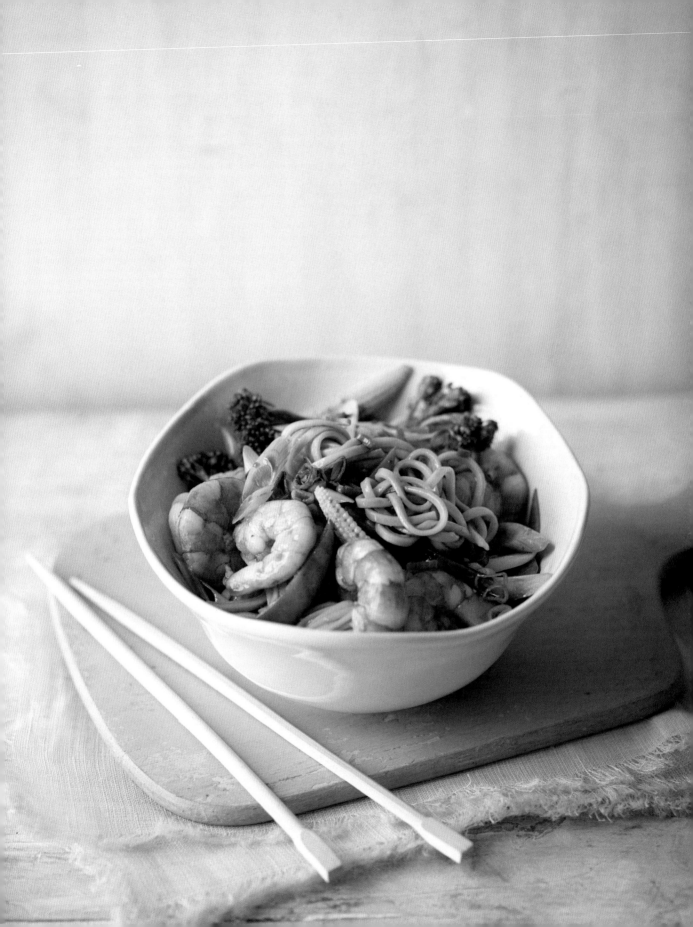

IN-A-HURRY CURRY FRIED RICE

SERVES 1

If you're craving a curry and thinking of ordering greasy takeout, hold your horses and make this instead. It's lean, it tastes great and it will arrive quicker than any Indian takeout. It tastes awesome with diced pork or turkey too.

MAKE AHEAD

INGREDIENTS

1 tbsp coconut oil
1 small red onion, roughly diced
1 clove garlic, roughly diced
¾ inch fresh ginger, roughly diced
½ lb boneless, skinless chicken breast, sliced into ⅓-inch-thick strips
½ red bell pepper, sliced
1 tbsp mild curry powder
9 oz pre-cooked basmati rice
big handful of baby spinach leaves
squeeze of lime juice

METHOD

Melt the coconut oil in a wok or large frying pan over medium to high heat. Add the onion and stir-fry for 1 minute, then add the garlic and ginger and cook for another minute. Toss in the chicken, bell pepper and half of the curry powder and stir-fry for 2 minutes.

Add the rice, crumbling it between your fingers as you drop it in, then pour in 2 tablespoons of water. Stir-fry for 2 minutes until the rice is warmed through and the chicken is completely cooked. Check by slicing into one of the larger pieces to make sure the meat is white all the way through, with no raw pink bits left.

Add the remaining curry powder, along with the spinach, and stir until the spinach has wilted slightly and the curry powder is evenly distributed.

Dish up your yummy curry fried rice, finishing with a big squeeze of lime juice.

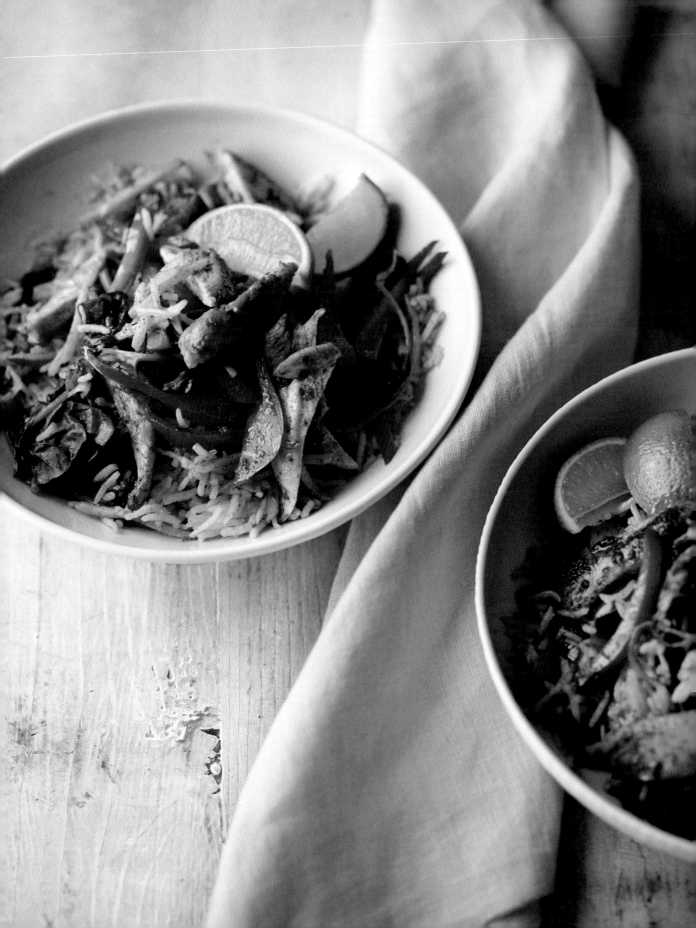

THE BODY COACH CLUB SANDWICH

SERVES 1

MAKE AHEAD
INGREDIENTS

2 eggs
salt and pepper
4 thick slices of bread
1 large tomato, sliced
½ head Bibb lettuce, leaves
only
10 oz mixed sliced deli-style
   meats—I like turkey and
   ham
1 big gherkin pickle, to serve
   —optional

The Body Coach club sandwich is a beautiful thing!
I've stuck with tradition and gone with turkey and ham,
but feel free to improvise. And if the four-layer sandwich
is too much for you, drop a layer and add a handful of
sweet potato fries instead (see Top Tip below).

METHOD

Bring a saucepan of water to a boil before carefully lowering in
the eggs and boiling for 6 minutes. Drain, then run the eggs
under cold water until cool enough to handle and peel them.
Place the eggs in a small bowl, season generously with salt and
pepper, then crush with the back of a fork.

Toast your bread. When the toast is ready, build up your
sandwich: lay the 4 slices of toast in front of you, spread each
one with the crushed egg, then divide the tomato, lettuce
and meat evenly among 3 of the slices. Stack up these 3 slices,
then flip the last one over to create a lid.

Slice into triangles and gobble down with a gherkin chaser.

★ TOP TIP

To make the sweet potato fries, slice a large sweet potato
lengthwise into 8 wedges. Microwave the wedges for
4 minutes, then let stand for 1 minute. Heat 1 tbsp of
coconut oil and fry the par-cooked fries in the oil until
browned and crisp all over. Drain on paper towels and
season with salt.

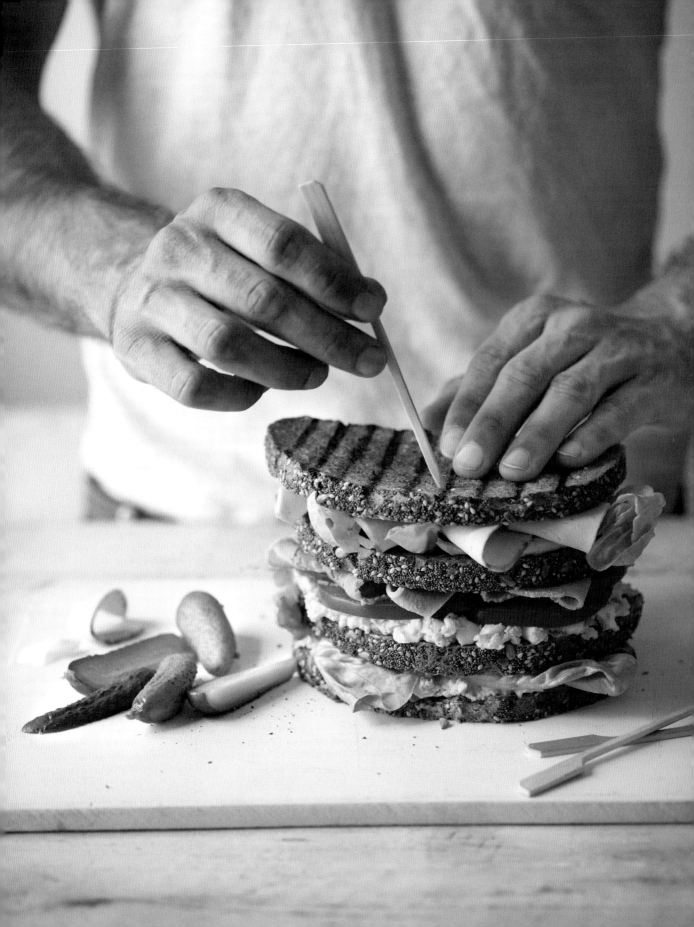

THAI BEEF STIR-FRY

SERVES 1

Fast and full of vibrant flavors, this will become a favorite. I predict you'll be eating this once a week when you've tried it. And if you become bored with egg noodles, try any of the "straight to wok" types, or choose rice noodles for a gluten-free meal.

MAKE AHEAD INGREDIENTS

½ tbsp coconut oil
2 star anise
1 bird's eye chile, finely
   chopped—remove the seeds
   if you don't like it hot
2 cloves garlic, finely chopped
3 scallions, finely sliced
1 lemongrass stalk, tender
   white part only, finely sliced
½ lb sirloin steak, trimmed
   of visible fat and sliced into
   ⅓-inch-thick strips
8 oz fresh egg noodles
2 tsp fish sauce
small bunch of cilantro,
   leaves only, roughly chopped
juice of 1 lime

METHOD

Melt the coconut oil in a wok or large frying pan over high heat. Add the star anise and let them infuse the oil for 30 seconds, then remove. Add the chile, garlic, scallions and lemongrass and stir-fry for 1 minute.

Add the steak and stir-fry for another 1–2 minutes until the beef is almost cooked.

Tumble in the noodles, along with a couple of tablespoons of water—this will create steam, helping to separate and warm the egg noodles. Toss everything together until you are satisfied that the beef is cooked and the noodles are warmed through.

Remove from the heat, add the fish sauce, cilantro and lime juice, then serve up.

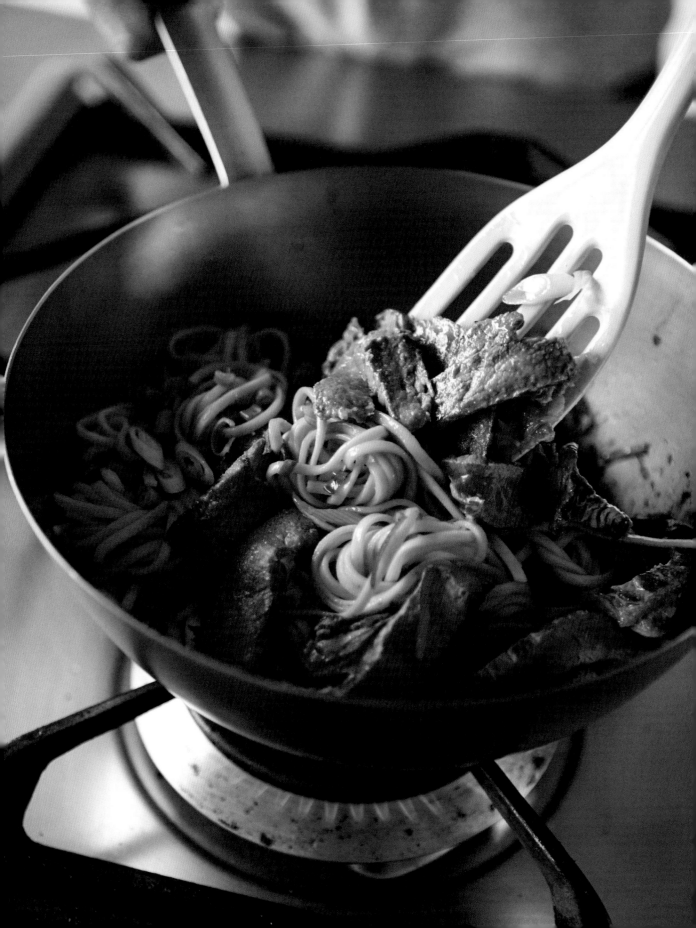

BAHN MI (VIETNAMESE PORK SANDWICH)

This Vietnamese speciality uses pork loin, which is a great source of low-fat, inexpensive protein.

SERVES 1

MAKE AHEAD
INGREDIENTS

½ tbsp coconut oil

½ red onion, sliced into thin wedges

10 oz boneless pork loin chops, cut into ⅓-inch-thick slices

1 red chile, sliced—remove the seeds if you don't like it hot

1 tbsp fish sauce

juice of 2 limes

2 tsp honey

2 tsp sesame oil

½ large baguette

1 tbsp chipotle paste

1 baby gem lettuce, leaves separated

¼ cucumber, sliced into thin matchsticks

mint and cilantro leaves, to serve

METHOD

Melt the coconut oil in a wok or frying pan over medium to high heat. Add the onion and fry for 2 minutes or until starting to soften. Increase the heat to high, add the pork and chile and stir-fry for 2–3 minutes, by which time the pork should be cooked through. Check by cutting into one of the larger pieces of meat to make sure there is no pink left. Remove the pan from the heat and pour in the fish sauce, lime juice, honey and sesame oil. Toss everything together until well mixed.

Cut the baguette in half lengthwise and spread evenly with the chipotle paste. Build up your sandwich by laying lettuce leaves on the base, followed by the pork, cucumber and fresh herbs. Clamp the other half of the baguette on top and devour it.

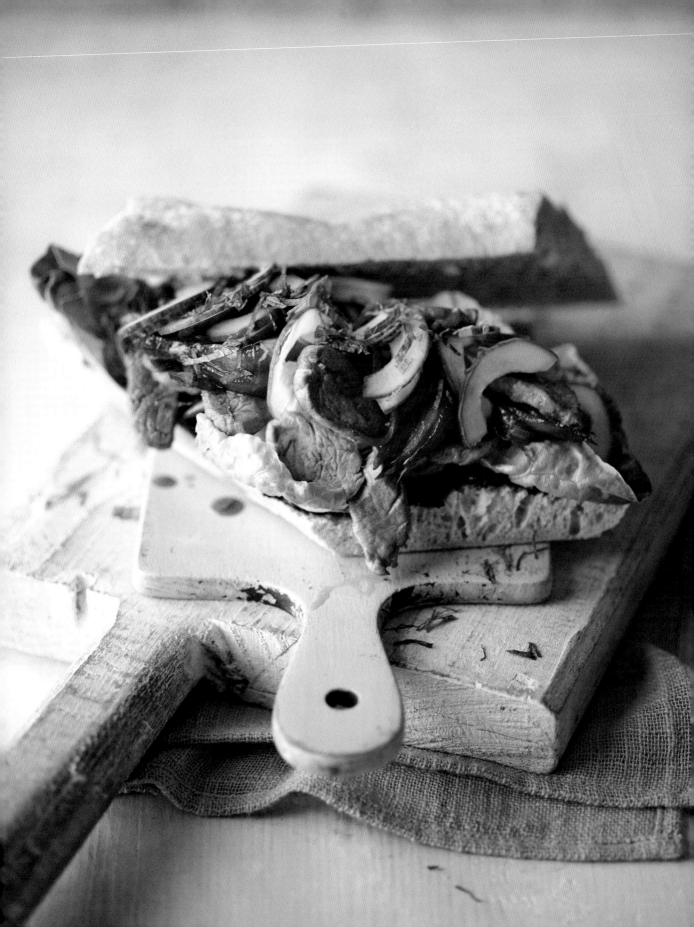

SERVES 1

SAG ALOO WITH CHICKEN

Potatoes don't need to be bland and boring. This Indian-inspired dish tastes incredible and is much leaner than greasy takeout from your local Indian restaurant.

MAKE AHEAD

INGREDIENTS

9 oz new potatoes
½ tbsp coconut oil
4 scallions, finely sliced
2 cloves garlic, finely chopped
¾ inch fresh ginger, finely
   chopped
1 tbsp garam masala
½ lb boneless, skinless
   chicken breast, sliced into
   ⅓-inch-thick strips
salt and pepper
2 large handfuls of baby
   spinach leaves
½ bunch of cilantro, leaves
   only, roughly chopped
squeeze of lemon juice

METHOD

Prick each potato once with a fork. Place in a microwaveable bowl, pour over a splash of water and microwave for 2½ minutes, then let rest for 30 seconds before giving them a final 3-minute blast. Let the potatoes stand for another 30 seconds, before carefully slicing them in half.

Melt the coconut oil in a wok or large frying pan over medium to high heat. Add the scallions, garlic and ginger and fry for 1 minute, stirring regularly. Tumble in the potatoes and mix in well. Sprinkle in the garam masala and fry for 30 seconds, stirring constantly—be careful not to let it stick. Quickly add the chicken, along with 2 tablespoons of water, to help cook the chicken and stop the spices burning. Season generously with salt and pepper and fry for 3–4 minutes, by which time the chicken should be cooked through. Check by slicing into one of the larger pieces to make sure the meat is white all the way through, with no raw pink bits left.

Add the spinach and toss through until wilted—there is no such thing as too much spinach at this point! Remove from the heat, sprinkle in the cilantro and finish with a squeeze of lemon juice.

TURKEY AND CHICKPEA PITAS

The flavors in this dish remind me of falafel. If you don't have chickpeas, try making it with cannellini or lima beans. And, if you like, you can ditch the pita and wrap it all up in a tortilla instead!

MAKE AHEAD

INGREDIENTS

1¼ cups canned chickpeas, drained and rinsed
½ tbsp coconut oil
½ red onion, diced
1 clove garlic, finely diced
9 oz ground turkey
2 tsp ground cumin
1 tsp smoked paprika
salt and pepper
1 carrot, grated
1 red chile, finely sliced—remove the seeds if you don't like it hot
½ bunch of cilantro, leaves only, roughly chopped
squeeze of lemon juice
2 pita breads, to serve

METHOD

Bring a saucepan of water to a boil, add the chickpeas and simmer for 5 minutes. Drain in a sieve or colander, then rinse under cold running water.

Meanwhile, heat the coconut oil in a large frying pan over high heat. Add the onion and garlic and fry for 1 minute, then throw in the turkey and fry for 2 minutes, breaking up any big lumps as you go. Sprinkle in the cumin and paprika and fry for 30 seconds, by which time the turkey should be cooked. Season generously with salt and pepper, then stir in the carrot, chile and chickpeas, using the back of your spoon to crush some of the chickpeas.

When you are happy that the turkey is fully cooked and the chickpeas are warmed through, remove the pan from the heat, stir through the chopped cilantro and finish with a good squeeze of lemon juice. Load into pita breads and eat.

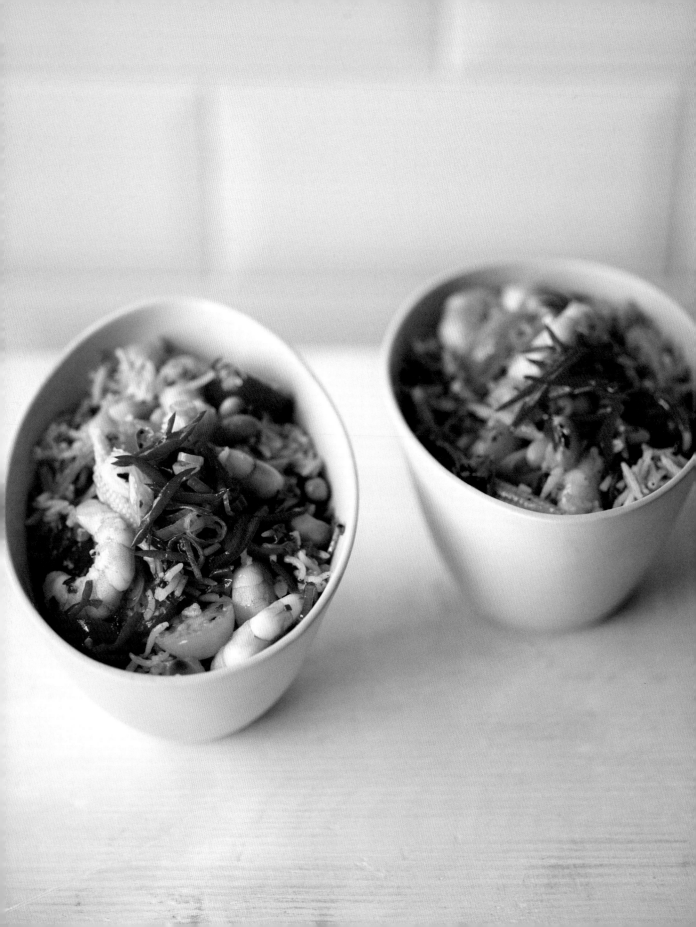

PIRI PIRI RICE WITH GARLIC SHRIMP

SERVES 1

I'm a massive fan of piri piri. It's one of my favorite seasonings and tastes awesome on most things. The black-eyed peas in this recipe add an extra protein boost. This is a great dish to double up, so you'll have some for lunch or dinner the next day.

METHOD

Heat half of the coconut oil in a wok or large frying pan over high heat. Add the scallions, chile, corn and tomato and stir-fry for about 1 minute. Add the piri piri seasoning and stir-fry for 30 seconds, then add the black-eyed peas, along with 2 tablespoons of water. Add the rice, crumbling it between your fingers as you drop it in, then stir-fry for about 2 minutes, breaking up any clumps with a wooden spoon. Add the spinach, giving it a couple of turns to help it wilt. Tip the rice and vegetables onto a plate and wipe out your frying pan.

Return the wok or pan to a high heat and add the rest of the coconut oil. When it is melted and hot, add the garlic and shrimp and cook for about 1 minute, stirring every now and then, until the shrimp are pink and cooked through.

Spoon the garlicky shrimp over the piri piri rice, finish with a squeeze of lemon juice and eat up.

MAKE AHEAD

INGREDIENTS

1 tbsp coconut oil
2 scallions, roughly chopped
1 red chile, roughly chopped—
  remove the seeds if you
  don't like it hot
6 baby corn, cut in half
4 cherry tomatoes, cut in half
2 tsp piri piri seasoning
½ cup canned black-eyed
  peas, drained and rinsed
5 oz pre-cooked rice
large handful of baby spinach
  leaves
1 large clove garlic, chopped
12 raw shrimp (about 7 oz),
  peeled
squeeze of lemon juice

SINGAPORE NOODLES

When you finish a workout feeling ravenous, you want food, and you want it fast. This is the dish for such times. It might seem like a strange combination, but the chicken, curry powder and shrimp are a total winner. If you don't fancy the combo, feel free to use either chicken or shrimp—in which case, you'll need 9 oz chicken or 7 oz shrimp.

SERVES 1

MAKE AHEAD
INGREDIENTS

1 tbsp coconut oil
5 oz boneless, skinless chicken breast, sliced into ⅓-inch-thick strips
1 tbsp mild curry powder
8 shrimp, peeled
2 scallions, roughly chopped
1 red chile, roughly chopped— remove the seeds if you don't like it hot
1 clove garlic, roughly chopped
2 oz snow peas, cut in half
6 baby corn, cut in half
7 oz fresh egg noodles
salt and pepper
juice of 1 lime
¼ bunch of cilantro, leaves only, roughly chopped

METHOD

Heat the oil in a wok or large frying pan over high heat. Add the chicken and fry for 1 minute, turning it a couple of times. When the chicken is no longer pink, sprinkle half of the curry powder into the wok and stir to coat the chicken strips.

Throw in the shrimp and toss with the other ingredients. Add the scallions, chile, garlic, snow peas and corn and stir-fry for about 2 minutes or until the shrimp are pink and the chicken is cooked through. Check the chicken by slicing into one of the larger pieces to make sure the meat is white all the way through, with no raw pink bits left.

Add the noodles, along with about 2 tablespoons of water— this will help to loosen any ingredients that may have stuck to the wok or pan, as well as helping to separate the noodles.

Sprinkle in the rest of the curry powder and season generously with salt and pepper. Toss everything together before piling the noodles onto a plate, drizzling over the lime juice and finishing with the chopped cilantro.

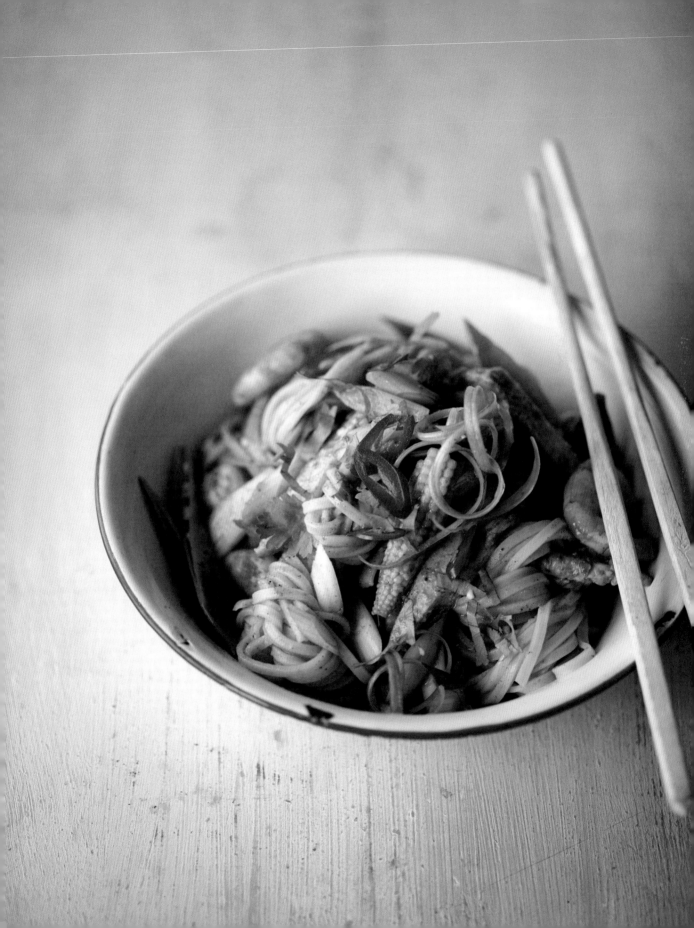

#BURGERME WITH SWEET POTATO FRIES

I'm sorry but I refuse to release a cookbook without at least a couple of healthy burger recipes. Burgers make me happy, and I promise this one won't disappoint. Stack it up like a boss and get it done!

INGREDIENTS

2 large sweet potatoes,
  cut into fries
1¼ lb 95% lean ground beef
1 small red onion, finely
  chopped
1 clove garlic, finely chopped
salt and pepper
1 tbsp coconut oil
2 tsp chipotle paste
2 tbsp crème fraîche
2 burger buns
1 tomato, sliced
2 gherkins, sliced
lettuce, to serve

METHOD

Preheat the broiler to high.

Zap the sweet potato fries in the microwave for 7 minutes, then let rest for 30 seconds.

While the sweet potato is spinning in the microwave, mix the beef with the onion and garlic—stick your hands in and work the ingredients together with a good pinch each of salt and pepper. Shape the mixture into two good-sized burgers about ¾ inch thick. Place on a broiler pan or a baking sheet and broil for 5 minutes on each side.

Heat the coconut oil in a large frying pan over high heat. Add the sweet potato fries and fry for about 3 minutes on each side or until they are nicely browned all over. Drain on paper towels, then season with a good pinch of salt.

Mix together the chipotle paste and crème fraîche in a small bowl.

Cut the burger buns in half, then build your burgers: start with a beef patty, then top with tomato, gherkins, lettuce and chipotle-crème fraiche sauce, finishing with the top half of the burger bun. Serve up with the sweet potato fries and shout out "Hashtag BurgerMe" just before you eat it.

SHRIMP, ZUCCHINI AND LENTIL CURRY

We usually think it takes ages to cook a curry, but some can be lightning quick to make! You can use chicken instead of shrimp if you want; even a bit of haddock would be good. And if you really want to mix it up, eggplant works as well as zucchini, though you'll need to cook it for a bit longer. Don't be afraid to use ready-made curry pastes, either—they are lifesavers!

MAKE AHEAD
GOOD TO FREEZE
INGREDIENTS

½ tbsp coconut oil
1 small red onion, diced
1 zucchini, diced
1 red chile, sliced—optional
1 tbsp curry paste—I like
  Patak's rogan josh or bhuna
¾ cup canned chopped
  tomatoes
10 oz raw shrimp, peeled
3½ oz pre-cooked Puy lentils
7 oz pre-cooked basmati rice
½ bunch of cilantro, leaves
  only, roughly chopped

METHOD

Melt the coconut oil in a wok or large frying pan over medium to high heat. Add the onion and zucchini—and the chile, if using—and stir-fry until starting to soften.

Spoon in the curry paste and fry for 30 seconds before pouring in the chopped tomatoes. Bring to a boil, then add the shrimp and lentils. Simmer the curry for 1 minute or until the lentils are warmed through and the shrimp are cooked—they're done when their flesh turns vibrant pink.

Meanwhile, zap your rice in the microwave, following the package instructions.

Stir the cilantro through your curry and serve up with the rice.

MIGHTY DUCK NOODLES

It's good to switch up your bird now and again. This quick and easy duck noodle dish makes a nice change from your standard chicken and turkey. The five-spice and hoisin create an absolute explosion of flavor.

MAKE AHEAD

INGREDIENTS

½ tbsp coconut oil

8 oz boneless duck breast,
  skin removed, sliced into
  ⅓-inch-thick strips

½ tsp five-spice powder

3 scallions, finely sliced

1 clove garlic, finely sliced

4 oz midget trees (broccolini),
  any bigger stalks sliced
  in half lengthwise

9 oz fresh egg noodles

2 tbsp hoisin sauce

¼ small cucumber, sliced into
  thin matchsticks

METHOD

Melt the coconut oil in a wok or large frying pan over medium to high heat. Add the duck and let it sizzle for a couple of minutes. When the duck is mostly browned, crank the heat up to high and add the five-spice powder, scallions, garlic and midget trees, along with about 2 tablespoons of water—this will steam up and help everything to cook. Stir-fry for about 3 minutes, then add the noodles, and toss until the noodles are warmed through.

Remove from the heat and pour in the hoisin sauce. Stir everything together into one delicious mass, then slide onto a plate and top with the cucumber.

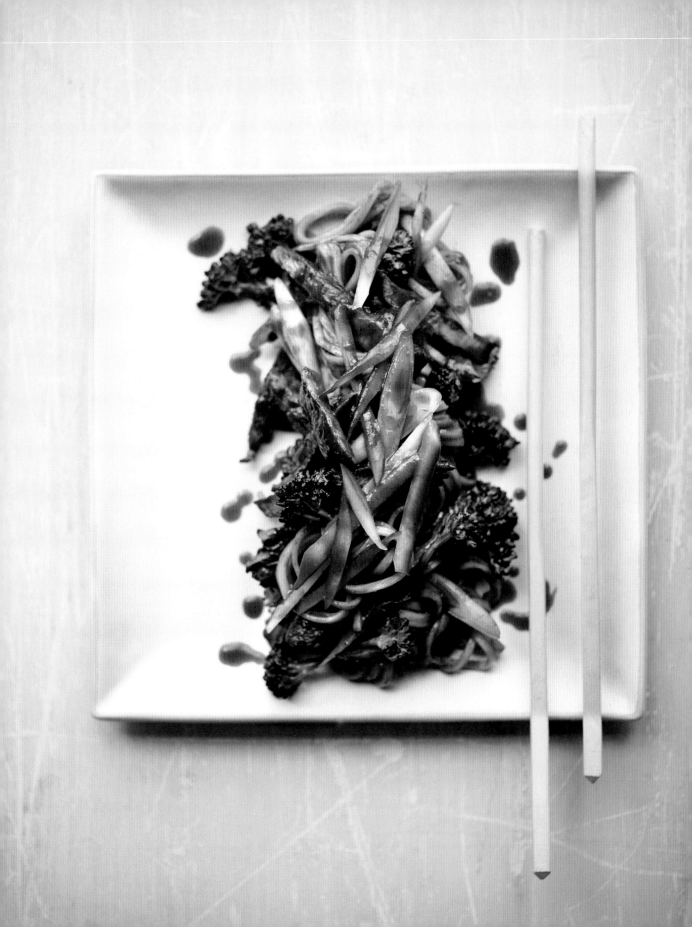

JOE'S McLEANIE BURGER

Another burger recipe? Guilty. Well, I did say I love burgers. And remember a turkey is not just for Thanksgiving—combined with all these tasty ingredients, you really won't be disappointed with this super-lean hero burger.

INGREDIENTS

14 oz ground turkey
1 tbsp fish sauce
½ bunch of cilantro, leaves only, roughly chopped
2 tsp sesame oil
4 scallions, finely sliced
salt and pepper
2 burger buns
2 tbsp full-fat Greek yogurt
1 tbsp chipotle paste
sliced tomato and lettuce leaves, to serve

METHOD

Preheat the broiler to high.

Chuck the turkey, fish sauce, cilantro, sesame oil and scallions into a large bowl. Season generously with salt and pepper, then stick your hands in and work the ingredients well. The more you work the meat, the better the burgers will hold together when cooked. Shape the meat into two equal patties.

Place the patties on a broiler pan or a baking sheet and broil the burgers for 5 minutes on each side or until they are totally cooked through. Check by slicing into one of the patties to make sure the meat is white all the way through, with no raw pink bits left.

Meanwhile, cut your burger buns in half. Mix together the yogurt and chipotle paste and spread over the burger buns.

When your burgers are cooked, remove from the broiler and build your dream burger, stacking it up with tomato and lettuce—the bigger, the better.

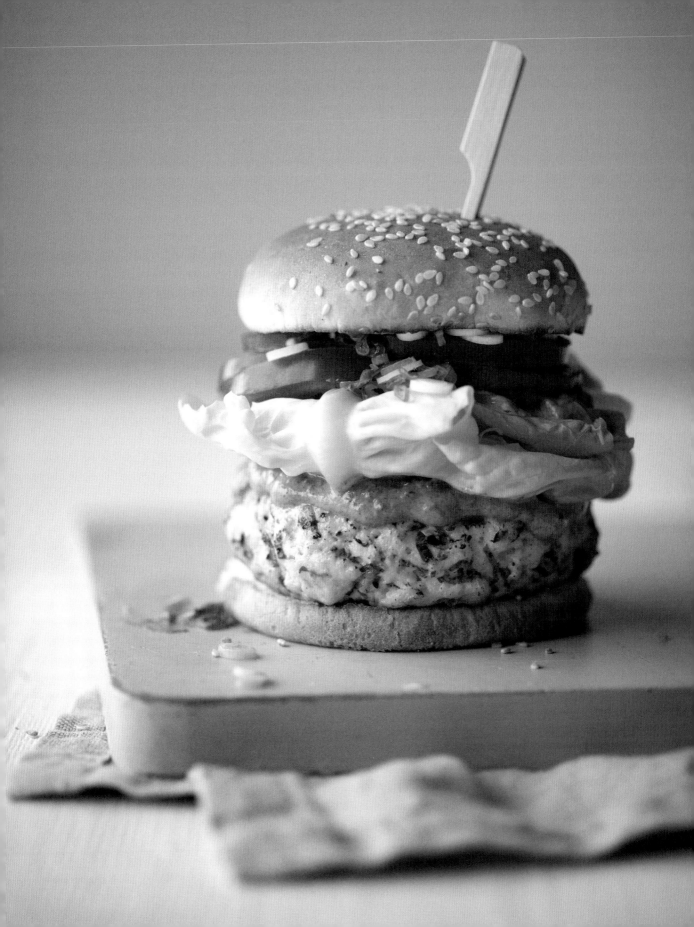

CHEEKY CHICKEN FRIED RICE

Do you ever just feel lazy and want to do as little work as possible in the kitchen? I do, and if you feel the same, then this one-wok, no-messing-about dish will be right up your alley. Pre-cooked, packaged rice is a great thing to have in the house for a quick meal—and for this, it doesn't even have to go in the microwave. Almost any vegetables can go into this fried rice, making it a great way of using up the stragglers. It's perfect for lunch the next day too, so you can always do a cheeky double-up with the recipe. #Guilty

SERVES 1

MAKE AHEAD
INGREDIENTS

1 tbsp coconut oil
1 clove garlic, finely chopped
⅓ inch fresh ginger, finely chopped
½ lb boneless, skinless chicken breast, sliced into ⅓-inch-thick strips
2 scallions, roughly chopped
1 carrot, chopped into ⅓-inch pieces
⅓ cup frozen peas
2 oz baby corn, roughly chopped
9 oz pre-cooked basmati rice
1 tbsp light soy sauce
2 tsp sesame oil
½ red chile, finely chopped—optional

METHOD

Melt the coconut oil in a wok or large frying pan over high heat. Throw in the garlic and ginger and stir-fry for 30 seconds.

Add the chicken and stir-fry for 2 minutes, by which time the chicken should have colored a little on the outside. Chuck in the scallions, carrot, peas and corn and stir-fry for another 2–3 minutes until the vegetables and chicken are cooked through. Check by slicing into one of the larger pieces of chicken to make sure the meat is white all the way through, with no raw pink bits left.

Tip in the rice straight from the package, along with about 1 tablespoon of water, and keep stir-frying for about 1 minute or until the rice is warmed through.

Remove the wok or pan from the heat and pour in the soy sauce and sesame oil. Top with red chile for added kick.

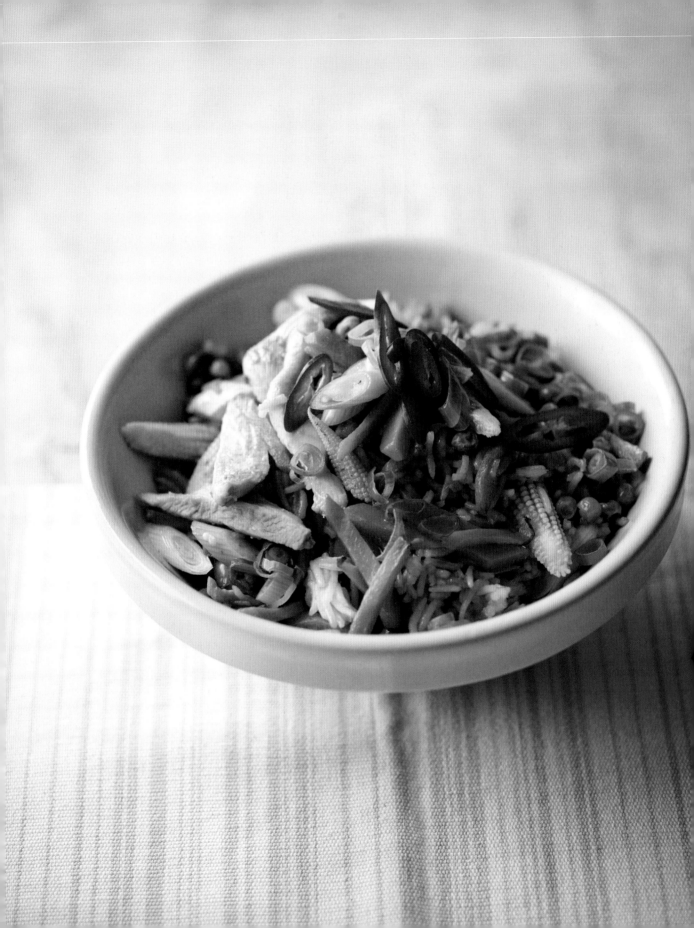

MAKE AHEAD
GOOD TO FREEZE
**(only the meatballs,
not the pasta)**
INGREDIENTS

**1 tbsp coconut oil
1 small red onion, diced
2 cloves garlic, finely chopped
2 sprigs of fresh thyme
1 can (14 oz) chopped
 tomatoes
12 (about 14 oz) ready-made
 turkey meatballs (or see
 page 93 to make your own)
2 large handfuls of baby
 spinach leaves
salt and pepper
14 oz fresh tagliatelle
½ bunch of basil, leaves only,
 roughly chopped**

MY BIG JUICY MEATBALLS AND PASTA

Yes, that's right, pasta! Don't be scared—you can eat pasta and still burn fat. This food mountain will leave you feeling like a champion when you clear the plate. Fresh pasta cuts down the cooking time, but isn't essential. And if you can't find turkey meatballs, pork or beef meatballs work just as well.

METHOD

Start by bringing a large saucepan of water to a boil, ready to cook the pasta.

In a large frying pan or another large saucepan, heat the coconut oil over medium to high heat. Add the onion, garlic and thyme to the pan and fry, stirring regularly, for 2 minutes or until the onion and garlic are just starting to soften. Pour in the tomatoes and bring to a boil. Carefully drop the meatballs into the sauce, then reduce the heat to a simmer and cover your pan with a lid. If you don't have a lid big enough, a large dinner plate or baking sheet should do the trick. Simmer the meatballs for about 6 minutes, or until cooked through. Check by cutting into one to make sure there are no raw pink bits of meat left. Add the spinach to the sauce and stir until wilted. Season with salt and pepper, then remove the pan from the heat.

Drop the tagliatelle into the boiling water and cook for about 2 minutes. Drain the pasta and tip it back into the pan. Spoon in about half of the meatballs and sauce and mix with the pasta. Divide the saucy pasta between two plates, spoon over the remaining sauce and garnish with the basil.

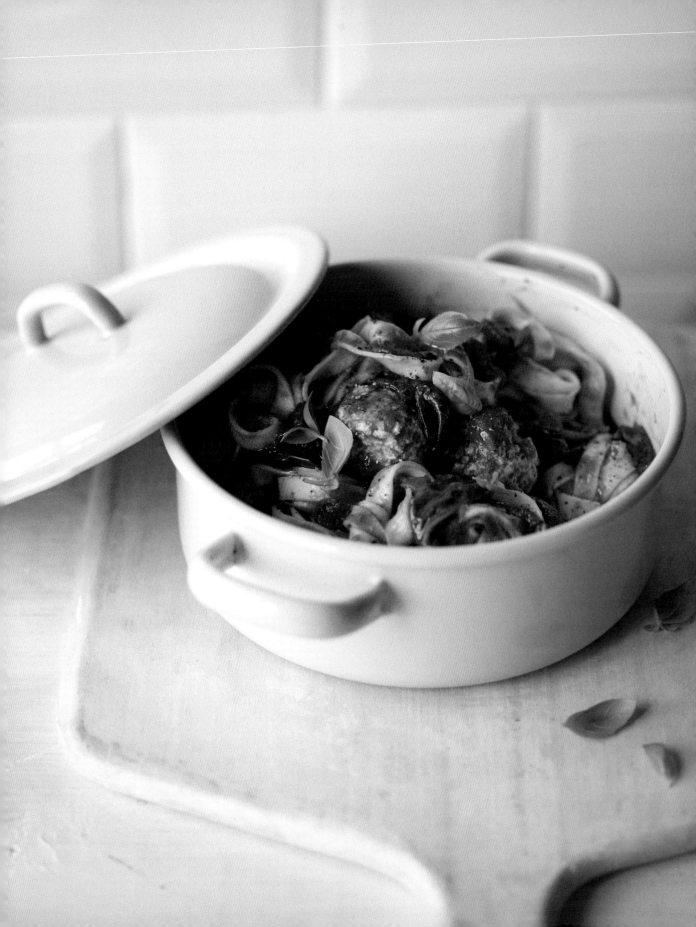

MAKE AHEAD
GOOD TO FREEZE
INGREDIENTS

½ tbsp coconut oil
2 scallions, finely sliced
10 oz smoked whitefish,
   skinned and cut into small
   chunks
1 zucchini, cut into ¾-inch
   cubes
¾ cup frozen peas
1 tbsp mild curry powder
1 egg
9 oz pre-cooked basmati rice
½ cup fat-free milk
large handful of baby spinach
   leaves
1 red chile, finely sliced—
   remove the seeds if you
   don't like it hot

KEDGEREE

This kedgeree (#weirdwordalert) tastes incredible—after a workout, it will refuel your body and satisfy your taste buds at the same time.

METHOD

Bring a saucepan of water to a boil, ready to poach the egg.

Melt the coconut oil in a large frying pan over medium to high heat. Add the scallions, smoked whitefish and zucchini and fry for 2–3 minutes, stirring regularly. Stir in the peas and cook until thawed, then sprinkle in the curry powder and cook for 1 minute.

This is a good time to carefully crack your egg into the hot water to poach. Cook the egg for about 4 minutes for a runny yolk, then carefully lift out with a slotted spoon and drain on paper towels.

While the egg is poaching, add the rice to the frying pan, crumbling it between your fingers as you drop it in, then stir-fry for a minute or two, breaking up any clumps with a wooden spoon. Pour in the milk and stir, then bring to the boil and simmer for about 30 seconds. Add the spinach and stir until wilted.

Pile the kedgeree onto a plate, top with the poached egg and scatter with sliced chile, then serve.

MAKE AHEAD
GOOD TO FREEZE

INGREDIENTS

1 tbsp olive oil
1 red onion, diced
1 clove garlic, chopped
1 sprig of rosemary
6 Italian sausages
1 tbsp balsamic vinegar
1 can (14 oz) chopped
   tomatoes
10 oz fresh gnocchi
½ bunch basil, leaves only,
   roughly chopped

GNOCCHI WITH SAUSAGE RAGU

This little Italian number is guaranteed to please. The gnocchi cook in no time, and the sausages are already full of flavor, making this a really tasty meal for very little effort.

METHOD

Bring a large saucepan of water to the boil, ready to cook the gnocchi.

In a frying pan, heat the olive oil over medium to high heat. Add the onion, garlic and rosemary and cook, stirring occasionally, for 2–3 minutes.

Taking one sausage at a time, squeeze tightly with your fingers about a third of the way along its length to force the meat from the sausage casing—a small ball of sausage meat should pop out of the end of the casing. Repeat the process until you have 18 balls of sausage meat. Discard the empty sausage casings.

Drop the balls of sausage meat into the frying pan, and gently tumble them around the pan to coat in the oil, onion and garlic. Crank up the heat to high and pour in the balsamic vinegar, then let it bubble away to almost nothing. Pour in the tomatoes, bring to a boil and simmer for 5–6 minutes.

Meanwhile, drop the gnocchi into the pan of boiling water and cook for about 2 minutes, or according to the package instructions, then drain.

Check that the balls of sausage meat are fully cooked through—cut into one to make sure—then divvy up the gnocchi, top with the sausage ragu and finish with the basil.

SAMMY THE SEA BASS WITH SPAGHETTI

You may notice on Instagram that I like to name my foods—and somehow Sammy the Sea Bass seems to fit this dish. You won't believe how easy this one is. The other great thing is that you can add any leftover veg from the fridge as well . . . But please don't forget to shout, "Bosh, midget trees" when you throw the broccoli in the pan!

**SERVES
1**

INGREDIENTS

3 oz dried spaghetti
½ tbsp olive oil
**2 skin-on sea bass fillets
(about 5 oz each)**
salt and pepper
**3 oz midget trees (broccolini),
any bigger stalks sliced
in half lengthwise**
**3 oz kale, thick stems
removed**
6 cherry tomatoes
**½ red chile, roughly sliced—
remove the seeds if you
don't like it hot**

METHOD

Bring a large saucepan of salted water to a boil. Drop in the spaghetti and let it cook for 2 minutes less than the time given on the package.

Meanwhile, heat the oil in a frying pan over medium heat. Season the sea bass with salt and pepper, and when the oil is hot, gently lay the fillets in the pan, skin side down, and fry for 2–3 minutes. Flip the fish over, remove the pan from the heat and let the fish cook in the residual heat for 2 minutes. Carefully lift the fish out of the pan, then peel off and discard the skin.

By now the spaghetti should be almost cooked. Throw in all of the veg, and simmer with the pasta for 2 minutes. The tomatoes may split a little, but don't worry. Drain the pasta and veg in a colander.

Take the pan used to fry the fish and place it back over medium to high heat. Tip in the spaghetti and veg, season generously with salt and pepper, and toss everything together for 1 minute—this final frying gives the dish extra flavor.

Spoon the spaghetti and vegetables into a shallow bowl, flake over the fish in large chunks and top with the sliced chile.

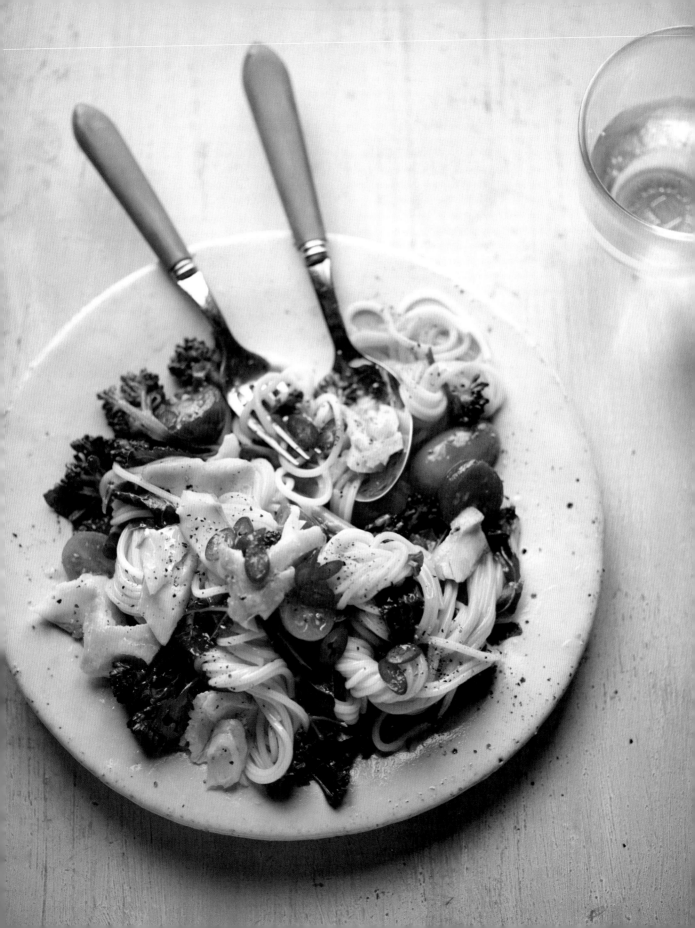

CHICKEN AND QUINOA STIR-FRY

**SERVES
1**

Quinoa used to be one of those obscure health foods, but these days it's everywhere—and luckily you can now get it pre-cooked in packages, so you don't have to wait 20 minutes for it to cook. The high protein content of quinoa makes this a great meal for building lean muscle.

MAKE AHEAD

INGREDIENTS

½ tbsp coconut oil
3 scallions, finely sliced
½ red bell pepper, finely diced
½ zucchini, diced
½ lb boneless, skinless chicken breast, cut into ⅓-inch-thick slices
2 tsp smoked paprika
salt and pepper
8 oz pre-cooked quinoa
1 oz feta, crumbled
small bunch of parsley, leaves only, roughly chopped —optional
squeeze of lemon juice

METHOD

Melt the coconut oil in a wok or large frying pan over medium to high heat. Add the scallions, bell pepper and zucchini and stir-fry for 2–3 minutes or until the vegetables are just starting to soften.

Increase the heat to high and add the chicken, along with the paprika and a little salt and pepper. Fry for another 3–4 minutes or until the chicken is just cooked. Check by slicing into one of the larger pieces to make sure the meat is white all the way through, with no raw pink bits left.

Stir in the quinoa and fry for a minute or so, until it is warmed through.

Serve your chicken and quinoa stir-fry topped with crumbled feta, chopped parsley (if using) and a squeeze of lemon juice.

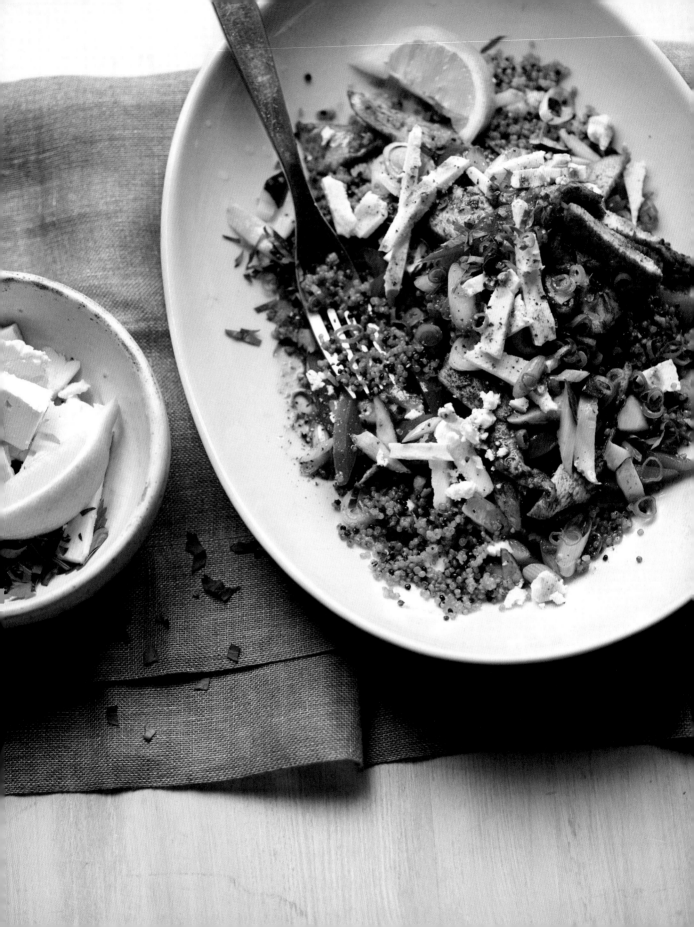

QUICK TORTILLA PIZZA

SERVES 1

This recipe is for all the pizza lovers out there. It may not have exactly the same effect as a cheesy stuffed-crust pizza, but it's cheaper, quicker and much leaner. Feel free to change the toppings and build your own dream pizza.

INGREDIENTS

4 large handfuls of baby spinach leaves

2 large tortillas

¾ cup canned chopped tomatoes

1 cup canned kidney beans, rinsed and drained

½ tsp dried oregano

8 black olives, pitted and cut in half

9 oz sliced cooked meat—I like ham or cold roast chicken

2 large eggs

salt and pepper

green salad, to serve—optional

METHOD

Put the kettle on to boil and preheat your oven to 450°F.

Tip the spinach into a large colander and pour over boiling water from the kettle until it wilts. Quickly run the spinach under cold water to cool, then use your hands to squeeze out as much moisture as possible.

Place the tortillas on a nonstick baking sheet. Mix together the tomatoes, kidney beans and oregano, then spread over the tortillas. Divide the wilted spinach evenly between the tortillas, then scatter over the olives and meat. Make a little well in the middle of each tortilla pizza and crack in an egg. Season the pizzas with salt and pepper, then slip into the hot oven and bake for 12 minutes, or until the edges are browned and the white of the egg is set.

Slide the pizzas onto a board and serve with a big green salad . . . or just wolf down.

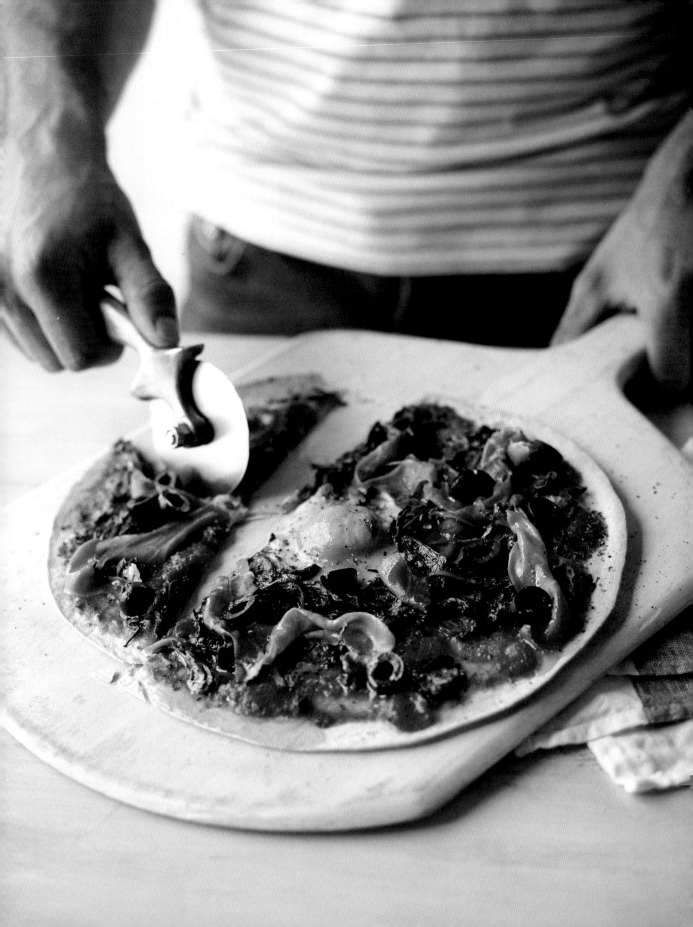

SPICED EGGPLANT AND CHICKPEAS WITH TURKEY

MAKE AHEAD
GOOD TO FREEZE
(the eggplant and chickpea stew, but not the turkey)

INGREDIENTS

1 tbsp coconut oil
4 scallions, cut into ⅓-inch
   slices
2 cloves garlic, finely sliced
1 small eggplant, cut into
   ⅓-inch dice
1 red chile, roughly chopped—
   remove the seeds if you
   don't like it hot
4 turkey cutlets (about 4 oz
   each
salt and pepper
1 tsp garam masala
1 tbsp tomato paste
1 can (15 oz) chickpeas,
   drained and rinsed
½ bunch of cilantro, leaves
   only, roughly chopped

Eggplant, chickpeas and Indian spices are a match made in heaven. This is a really hearty and filling post-workout meal. If you're not cooking for two, box up the rest and keep it in the fridge for tomorrow's lunch or dinner.

METHOD

Preheat the broiler to high.

Heat the coconut oil in a wok or large frying pan over medium to high heat. Add the scallions, garlic, eggplant and chile and stir-fry for 3–4 minutes.

While the vegetables are cooking, season the turkey steaks and broil them for 4–5 minutes on each side until cooked through. Check by cutting into the thickest part of one of the turkey steaks to make sure the meat is white all the way through, with no raw pink bits left. Remove and leave to rest.

Back to the vegetables in the wok or pan: add the garam masala and tomato paste and cook for a minute, stirring so the spices don't burn. Pour in ¾ cup of water, along with the chickpeas, then season generously with salt and pepper, bring to a simmer and cook for 2 minutes.

Serve up the chickpea and eggplant stew, then top with the turkey and finish with the cilantro.

SAUSAGE AND LENTIL CASSEROLE

MAKE AHEAD
GOOD TO FREEZE
INGREDIENTS

½ tbsp coconut oil
3 Italian sausages
1 red bell pepper, thinly
   sliced
½ zucchini, cut into
   ⅓-inch dice
10 cherry tomatoes
2 sprigs of thyme
9 oz pre-cooked Puy lentils
⅔ cup chicken stock
salt and pepper
½ bunch of parsley, leaves
   only, roughly chopped—
   optional

Don't worry, I know what you're thinking: how on earth can I make a casserole in 15 minutes? The secret to speeding this up is pre-cooked lentils. It tastes just as good as any 4-hour casserole, though, so give it a crack.

METHOD

Heat the coconut oil in a large frying pan over medium to high heat. Add the sausages and cook for 3 minutes to brown, turning them a couple of times.

Add the bell pepper, zucchini, tomatoes and thyme and stir-fry for 3–4 minutes or until the vegetables are just starting to soften. Tip in the lentils, along with the stock, and season generously with salt and pepper. Mix everything together, bring to a simmer and cook for 3–4 minutes.

Make sure the lentils are hot and the sausages are cooked through, then scatter over the parsley, if using, and serve immediately.

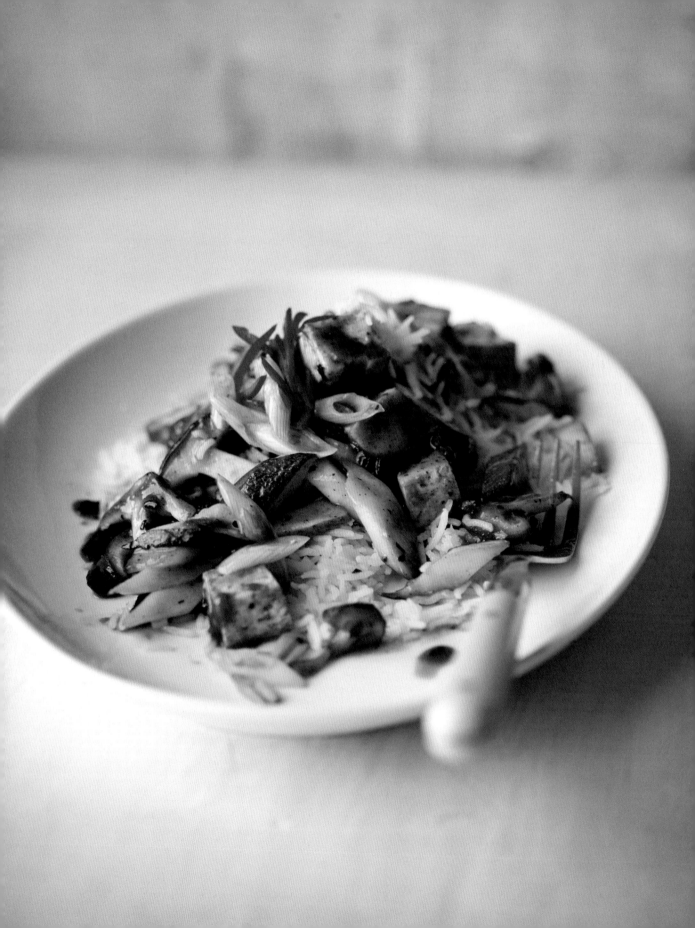

BLACK BEAN TOFU WITH SHIITAKE AND RICE

SERVES 2

MAKE AHEAD

INGREDIENTS

- 1 tbsp coconut oil
- 1 zucchini, cut into ⅓-inch dice
- 1 red chile, roughly chopped— remove the seeds if you don't like it hot
- 2 cloves garlic, roughly chopped
- 6 scallions, cut into ⅓-inch slices
- 8 shiitake mushrooms, roughly chopped
- 2 tbsp black bean sauce
- 14 oz firm tofu, cut into ¾-inch cubes
- 9 oz pre-cooked jasmine or basmati rice

I do apologize for the lack of veggie recipes, but I'm a meat-lover myself! Here's one that vegetarians, meat eaters and pescatarians will all love, though. When cooked with the right ingredients and flavors, tofu is really tasty—and if you eat a big enough portion, you can get a decent protein hit.

METHOD

Heat the coconut oil in a wok or large frying pan over medium to high heat. Throw in the zucchini and stir-fry for 1 minute. Add the chile, garlic, scallions and shiitake and stir-fry for 3–4 minutes, or until all the vegetables are starting to soften.

Spoon in the black bean sauce and pour in ⅔ cup of water. Bring to a simmer, then drop in the tofu and simmer gently for about 2 minutes or until heated through.

Zap your rice in the microwave and divide it between two plates, then top with the spicy, rich tofu.

TERIYAKI CHICKEN STIR-FRY

This is one of those dishes you'll love so much you'll want to make it every day. You can just walk in from work and smash this all in a wok, with little mess to clean up afterward—a true Lean in 15 recipe.

SERVES 1

MAKE AHEAD
INGREDIENTS

½ tbsp coconut oil
3 scallions, finely sliced
2 cloves garlic, finely sliced
¾ inch fresh ginger, finely chopped or grated
½ lb boneless, skinless chicken breast, sliced into ⅓-inch-thick strips
2 heads of bok choy, leaves separated
8 oz fresh egg noodles
large handful of baby spinach leaves
½ tbsp honey
1 tbsp light soy sauce
2 tsp rice wine vinegar
1 red chile, finely sliced—remove the seeds if you don't like it hot

METHOD

Heat the coconut oil in a wok or large frying pan over high heat. Add the scallions, garlic and ginger and stir-fry for 10 seconds, then add the chicken and stir-fry for 1 minute.

Throw in the bok choy, noodles, spinach and a couple of tablespoons of water—this will create steam to help cook the vegetables and separate the noodles. Stir-fry for 2–3 minutes, by which time the vegetables will have wilted and the chicken should be totally cooked through. Check by slicing into one of the larger pieces to make sure the meat is white all the way through, with no raw pink bits left.

Remove from the heat and pour in the honey, soy sauce and vinegar, mixing well. Pile the stir-fry onto a plate, top with the sliced chile and get it down you.

★ TOP TIP

If you can't find fresh egg noodles, just use dried ones—but remember they'll need rehydrating before you add them to the stir-fry. And for a gluten-free meal, swap the soy sauce for tamari, and use rice noodles instead of egg noodles.

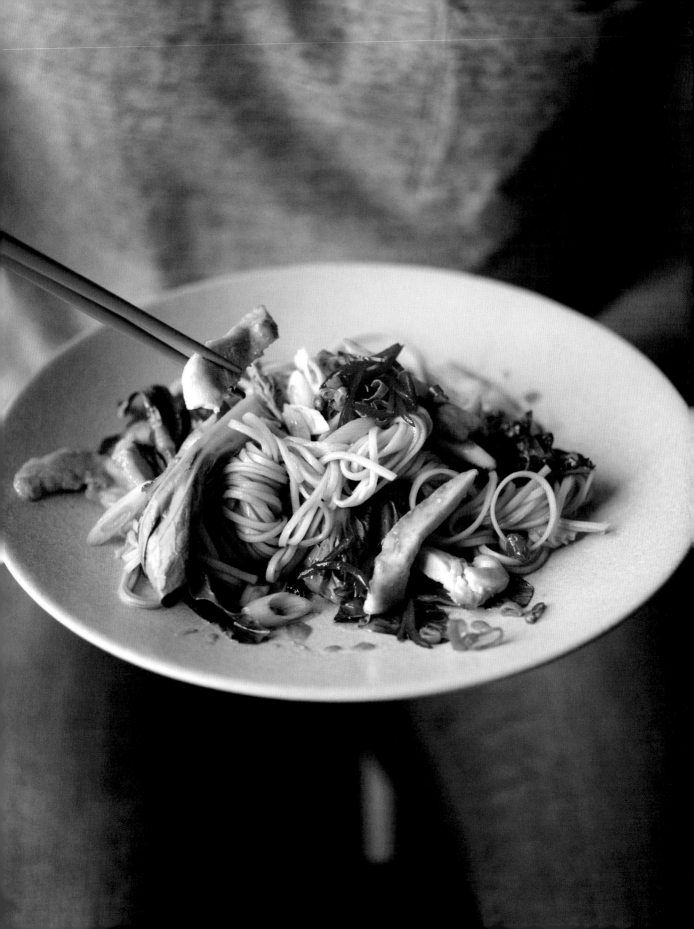

MAKE AHEAD
INGREDIENTS

½ lb boneless, skinless
  chicken breast
salt and pepper
1 tbsp ketchup
½ tsp smoked paprika
1 tbsp Worcestershire sauce
2 large tortilla wraps
1 baby gem lettuce, shredded
6 cherry tomatoes, halved
¼ cup canned black-eyed
  peas, drained and rinsed
2 tbsp cottage cheese

BIG BARBECUE CHICKEN WRAP

This easy chicken wrap with barbecue sauce goes down
a treat after a workout. Wrapped up tightly in foil, it's the
ideal lunch on the go.

METHOD

Preheat the broiler to high.

Spread out a large piece of plastic wrap on your cutting board
or counter. Lay the chicken on the plastic wrap and place
another piece of plastic wrap on top. Using a rolling pin, heavy
saucepan or any other blunt object, bash the chicken until
it is at least half its original thickness.

Remove the chicken from the plastic wrap and season with
salt and pepper, then place on a broiler pan or a baking sheet
and broil for 4 minutes, without turning.

Meanwhile, mix together the ketchup, paprika and
Worcestershire sauce until you have a smooth barbecue sauce.
Flip the chicken over and give it 2 more minutes, then smear
over a little of the sauce and broil for another 3–4 minutes,
or until it is fully cooked through. Check by slicing into it to
make sure the meat is white all the way through, with no raw
pink bits left.

Slice the cooked chicken into long strips. Spread the remaining
barbecue sauce over the tortillas, then top with the chicken,
lettuce, tomatoes, beans and cottage cheese. Roll up your big fat
tortillas and get munching.

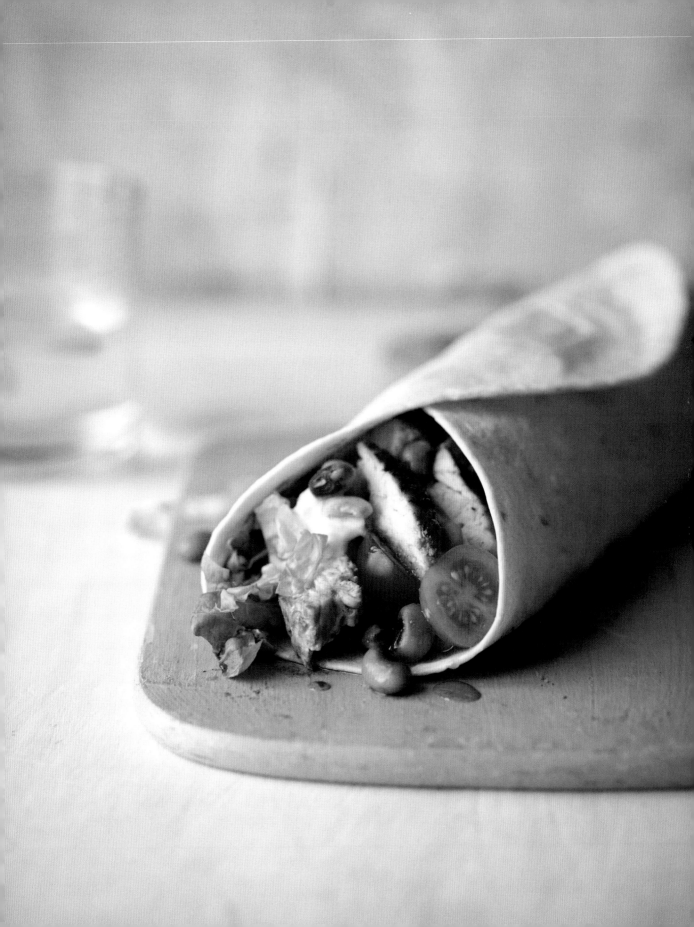

TOMATO DAAL WITH CHICKEN

Clocking in at about an hour, this is another recipe that takes longer than 15 minutes. Don't be put off, though—it's full of flavor and really satisfying after a workout, so it's worth the wait. If you're after a shortcut, batch-cook the daal and freeze the extra, ready for the next time.

LONGER RECIPE
MAKE AHEAD
GOOD TO FREEZE

INGREDIENTS

¾ cup yellow split peas
1½ tbsp coconut oil
1 tsp cumin seeds
1 fresh bay leaf, or 2 dried
1 large red onion, diced
4 cloves garlic, finely chopped
2 red chiles, diced—remove
  the seeds if you don't like
  it hot
2 inches fresh ginger, diced
½ tsp ground turmeric
1 tbsp garam masala
5 large tomatoes, roughly
  chopped
1 cup chicken stock
1¼ lb boneless, skinless
  chicken breast, sliced into
  ⅓-inch strips
salt and pepper
bunch of cilantro, leaves
  only, roughly chopped

METHOD

Tip the split peas into a large bowl and cover with warm water from the tap, then let soak for at least 20 minutes.

Melt 1 tablespoon of the coconut oil in a large saucepan over medium to high heat. Add the cumin seeds and bay leaf and fry for 30 seconds, then add the onion and stir-fry for 2–3 minutes or until just starting to soften and brown. Drop in the garlic, chiles and ginger and stir-fry for 1 minute.

Sprinkle in the turmeric and the garam masala and stir constantly for 30 seconds. Chuck in the tomatoes and chicken stock, then bring to a boil. Drain and rinse the soaked split peas and add them to the pan. Simmer for about 40 minutes, stirring regularly, and adding a little extra water if necessary, by which time the split peas should be completely cooked and starting to fall apart.

When the daal is nearly ready, melt the remaining coconut oil in a frying pan and add the chicken, seasoning it generously with salt and pepper. Fry for about 3 minutes or until the chicken is cooked through. Check by slicing into one of the larger pieces to make sure the meat is white all the way through, with no raw pink bits left.

Stir the cilantro through the cooked daal, top with the chicken and serve.

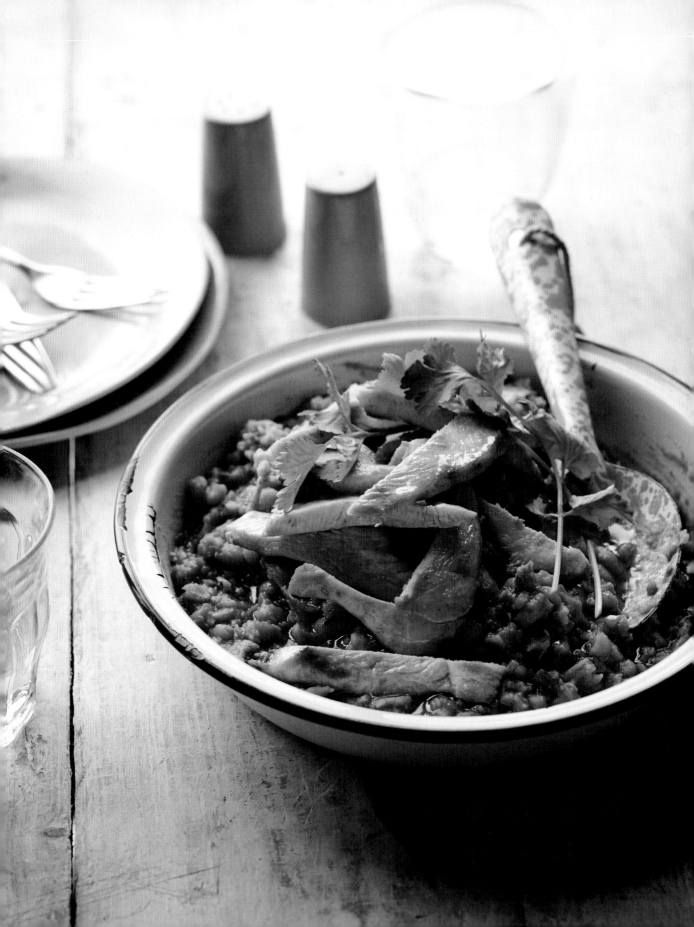

LONGER RECIPE
MAKE AHEAD
GOOD TO FREEZE

INGREDIENTS

1½ tbsp olive oil
2¼ lb 95% lean ground beef
1 large red onion, diced
1 carrot, diced
1 zucchini, diced
2 cloves garlic, finely chopped
1 tbsp tomato paste
1⅔ cups beef stock
1 can (14 oz) chopped
  tomatoes
18 no-boil lasagna sheets
bunch of basil, leaves only,
  roughly torn—optional
crusty bread, to serve

MY MUM'S SPECIAL LASAGNA

This is my mum's special recipe. In fact, as she would say, it's
the only thing she can cook. She's Italian, and when she was
growing up, she used to make this almost every week. Being
a lasagna, it takes more like an hour and 15 minutes from start
to finish, but it doesn't take too long to prep—and once it's in
the oven you can sit back and relax. I'm sure you will love this,
just like I always have.

METHOD

Heat ½ tablespoon of the olive oil in a large saucepan over
high heat. Add half the beef and fry for 2–3 minutes, stirring
to break up the chunks. Tip out onto a plate, then repeat with
another ½ tablespoon of oil and the rest of the beef.

When the meat has all been browned, wipe out your pan and
heat the remaining ½ tablespoon of oil over medium to high
heat. Add the onion, carrot, zucchini and garlic and cook,
stirring regularly, for about 5 minutes—by which time the
vegetables should have started to soften and color a little.
Add the tomato paste, beef stock and tomatoes, then return
the beef to the pan. Bring to a simmer and cook for 20 minutes.

Preheat the oven to 375°F.

Start building your lasagna in a 12 × 6-inch baking dish. Spoon
in about a quarter of the meat sauce, spreading it over the
bottom of the dish, then lay 6 sheets of pasta on top (don't
worry too much if they overlap). Repeat the process until you
have four layers of meat sauce and three layers of pasta—your
last layer should be a layer of meat sauce. Tightly cover the
dish with foil and bake in the oven for 40 minutes, or until it is
heated through and the pasta is fully cooked—you should be
able to easily insert a fork into the lasagna.

Finish the lasagna with a scattering of freshly torn basil, if you
like, and serve with a chunk of bread and a green salad.

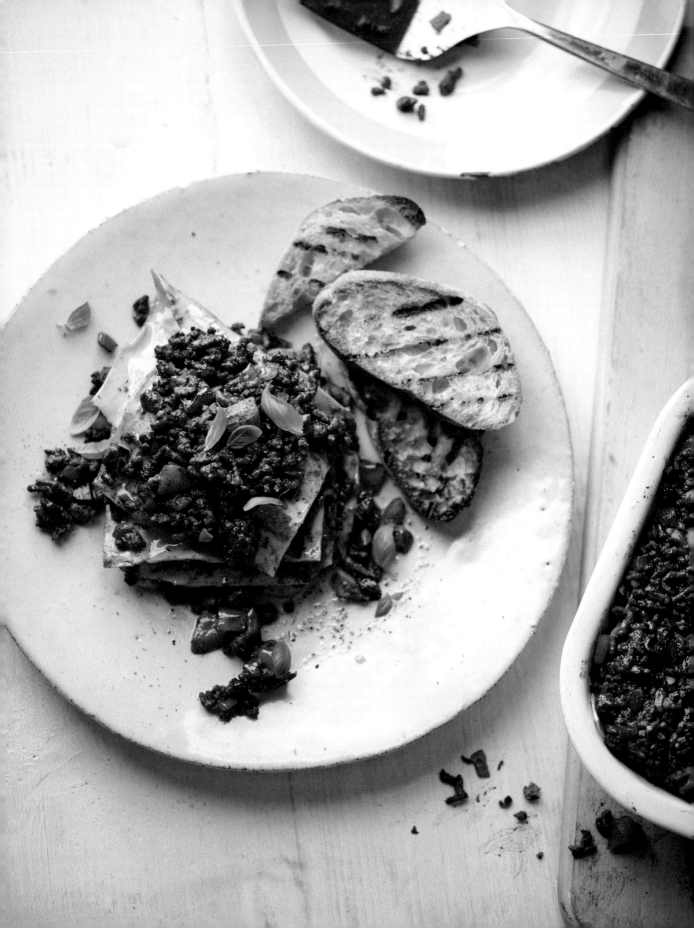

LONGER RECIPE
MAKE AHEAD
INGREDIENTS

**12 new potatoes
1 tbsp olive oil
5 scallions, sliced
1 red chile, thinly sliced—
 remove the seeds if you
 don't like it hot
2 handfuls of baby spinach
 leaves, plus a little extra to
 serve
10 oz deli-style cooked
 chicken or ham, roughly
 torn or sliced
8 eggs
salt and pepper
bread, to serve
cherry tomatoes, to serve**

SPANISH OMELETTE

This super-satisfying potato omelette needs about 30 minutes of your time, but it tastes great hot or cold, and so is perfect for carrying in a lunch box to work with some fresh salad.

METHOD

Prick the potatoes with a fork and microwave for 3 minutes. Let them rest for 2 minutes, then blast them for another 2 minutes, by which time they should be cooked through. Let cool and then slice them up.

Preheat the broiler to high.

Heat the olive oil in a nonstick frying pan (about 8 inches in diameter) over medium to high heat. Add the potatoes, and fry, turning every now and then, for 2 minutes. Add the scallions and chile and cook for another minute. Throw in the spinach, along with the chicken or ham, and fry for about 30 seconds or until the spinach has wilted.

Beat the eggs with a good pinch of salt and pepper, then pour into the frying pan. Use a wooden spoon or spatula to move the egg around, scraping it up from the bottom, for 1–2 minutes or until there is a good proportion of cooked egg in the pan. Leave the egg to cook for a minute longer, then slide the pan under the broiler (if your frying pan has a plastic handle, make sure that this doesn't go under the broiler!) and cook until the top of the omelette is just set.

Slide your omelette from the pan and cut it in half, then serve with a good chunk of bread and a side salad of the cherry tomatoes and the extra spinach.

LONGER RECIPE
GOOD TO FREEZE
INGREDIENTS

4 sweet potatoes, peeled and
   cut into chunks
salt and pepper
1 tbsp coconut oil
2¼ lb 95% lean ground beef
1 onion, roughly diced
1 red pepper, diced
2 carrots, grated
1 zucchini, grated
2 tbsp tomato paste
1 cup beef stock
generous ½ cup frozen peas
3 tbsp Worcestershire sauce

JOE'S SWEET POTATO COTTAGE PIE

Trust me, this dish takes a little while to cook (about 1 hour and 15 minutes), but the prep is easy and once you bang it in the oven, all you need is patience! The sweet potato topping makes this a real winner.

METHOD

Preheat your oven to 400°F.

Bring a large saucepan of water to a boil. Add the sweet potato and simmer for about 10 minutes or until very tender. Drain in a colander, give them a little shake to get rid of some of the moisture, then tip back into the pan. Season generously with salt and pepper, then mash until reasonably smooth.

While the sweet potatoes are cooking, heat half of the coconut oil in a large frying pan or heavy-bottomed pot over high heat. Add the ground beef and fry, breaking up any chunks, until the meat is just cooked and browned in places. Depending on the size of your pan, you may need to do this in two batches. Transfer the cooked meat to a bowl.

Heat the rest of the coconut oil in the same pan over medium to high heat. Add the onion, bell pepper, carrots and zucchini and stir-fry for 5–6 minutes or until they just begin to soften. Add the tomato paste and cook, stirring, for another 30 seconds, then tip the meat back in and stir well. Pour in the stock, bring to a boil and simmer for 20 minutes.

Remove from the heat and stir in the peas and Worcestershire sauce, then spoon into a large baking dish and top with the mashed sweet potato.

Bake your cottage pie for about 20 minutes, by which time the sweet potato topping should have crisped a little.

LONGER RECIPE
MAKE AHEAD
GOOD TO FREEZE

INGREDIENTS

1½ tbsp olive oil
1 large red onion, diced
3 cloves garlic, finely chopped
2¼ lb ground turkey
3 large handfuls of baby
  spinach leaves
1¼ cups ricotta
salt and pepper
1 bunch of basil, leaves only,
  roughly chopped
16 dried cannelloni tubes
2 cans (14 oz each) chopped
  tomatoes
crusty bread and a side salad,
  to serve

SPINACH AND TURKEY CANNELLONI

This is another batch-cooking winner. Invest an hour and 15 minutes of your time, then divide your cannelloni into 4 portions and you're all set for a few days. If you don't enjoy ground turkey, just use beef instead.

METHOD

Preheat the oven to 350°F.

Heat 1 tablespoon of the olive oil in a large frying pan over medium to high heat. Add the onion and garlic and fry for 2 minutes, stirring regularly, until the onions are soft and taking on a little color.

Increase the heat to high, add half of the turkey and fry for 2–3 minutes, breaking up any lumps with your spoon as you go. Cook the turkey until there is no more pink left, then tip out into a bowl. Repeat the process with the remaining olive oil and turkey. When this second batch is browned, toss the spinach into the pan and stir until wilted, then tip the whole lot into the bowl with the rest of the turkey.

Add the ricotta to the bowl, along with a generous amount of salt and pepper and half of the basil, and mix everything together well. Using your fingers and a teaspoon, stuff the cannelloni tubes with the turkey mixture—don't worry about being perfect here, any overspill can just be added into the sauce later.

When all of the tubes are full, pour one of the cans of tomatoes into the bottom of a large baking dish (about 12 × 7-inch) and stir in any leftover turkey mixture. Now line up the stuffed cannelloni tubes in the dish and pour over the second can of tomatoes, then cover the dish with foil.

Bake your cannelloni for 35–40 minutes, by which time the pasta should be cooked through. Remove from the oven, scatter with the rest of the basil and serve with a side salad and chunks of bread.

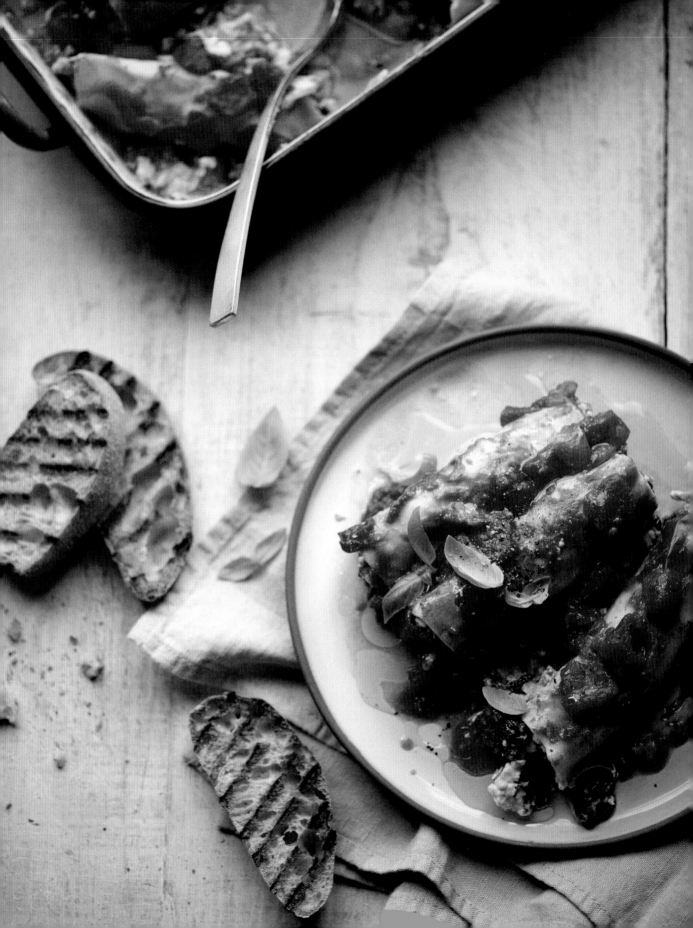

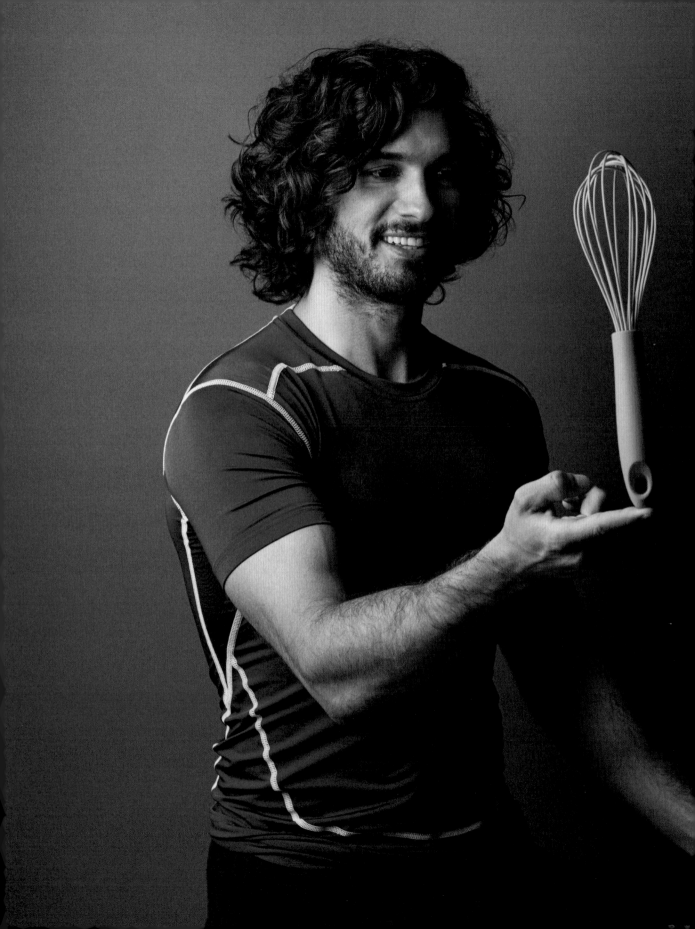

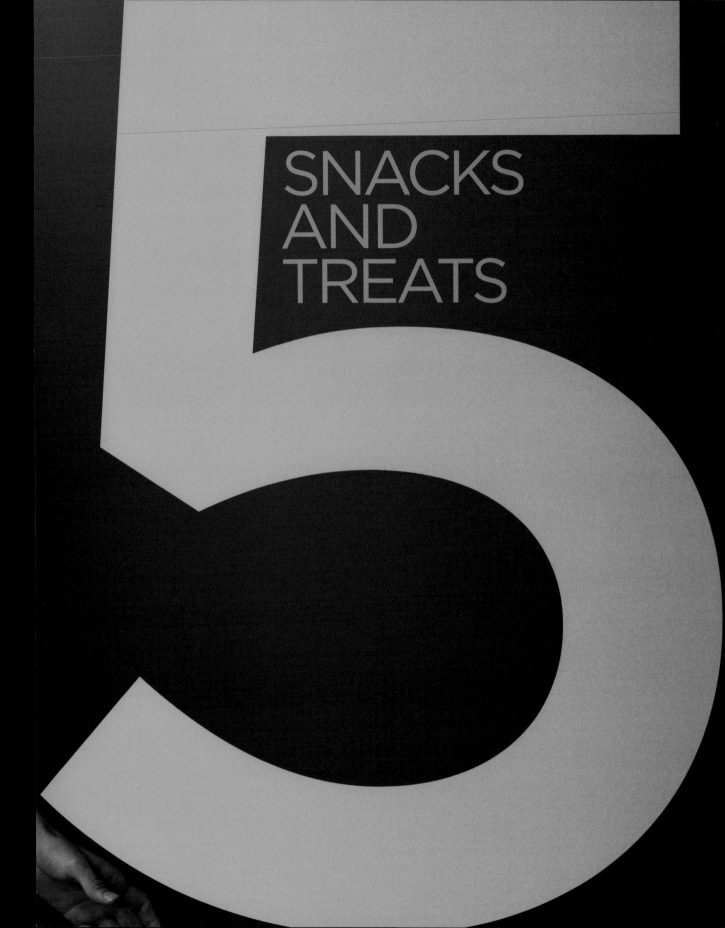

SNACKS AND TREATS

5

TUNA TARTARE

SERVES 2

If you like sushi, you will love this tartare. Good-quality fresh tuna should be fine to eat raw, but ask at your fishmonger or the fish counter in your local supermarket to be sure, letting them know you'll be eating the fish raw. Definitely give this dish a miss if you are pregnant or have a weakened immune system.

INGREDIENTS

¼ cup rice wine vinegar
1 tsp salt
½ cucumber, seeded and cut into ⅓-inch dice
14 oz raw tuna, cut into ⅓-inch dice—or smaller if you can
whole-grain rice cakes or rice crackers, to serve

METHOD

Pour the vinegar into a small bowl and thoroughly mix in the salt. Add the cucumber and let pickle for 5 minutes.

Drain off the vinegar and mix the lightly pickled cucumber with the tuna.

Serve up your raw fish treat with rice cakes or crackers for a delicious and different snack.

★ TOP TIP

You're working hard and training hard so why not treat yourself to one of my Lean in 15 treats? They're quite addictive, so don't get too greedy—share them with your friends! People are going to love you if you turn up to a party with healthy treats!

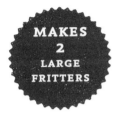

MAKE AHEAD
GOOD TO FREEZE
INGREDIENTS

1 can (12 oz) corn, drained
1 red chile, de-seeded and
   sliced, plus extra to serve—
   optional
3 scallions, finely sliced
2½ oz feta, crumbled
⅓ cup self-rising flour
1 egg
salt and pepper
1 tbsp coconut oil
1 avocado, sliced
juice of 1 lime, to serve
drizzle of sesame oil—
   optional

CORN AND FETA FRITTERS

These taste incredible and are very easy to make. They are good hot or cold, so you can make them the night before, ready to take to work in the morning. You can also double up the recipe and freeze half for another time.

METHOD

Place the corn, chile (if using), scallions, feta, flour, egg and ¼ cup of water in a large bowl. Season with salt and pepper, then mix until you have a lumpy batter.

Heat half of the coconut oil in a nonstick frying pan over low to medium heat. When the oil is hot, spoon in half of the batter, spreading it evenly around the pan. Cook the batter for about 2 minutes without flipping or budging . . . that's about time for 20 push-ups!

Flip the fritter and cook for another 2 minutes. Remove from the pan and transfer to paper towels to drain off any excess oil while you cook the second fritter.

Serve the fritters with the avocado, a good squeeze of lime juice and, if you like, a drizzle of sesame oil and a sprinkling of chile (see picture pg. 171).

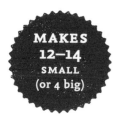

MAKE AHEAD
GOOD TO FREEZE

INGREDIENTS

1 can (5 oz) tuna, drained
1 zucchini, grated
⅔ cup self-rising flour
1 egg
1 tbsp coconut oil
light soy sauce, to serve

TUNA AND ZUCCHINI FRITTERS

Such an awesome and tasty snack—and there's nearly always a spare can of tuna knocking about in the pantry. You can batch-cook and freeze these too, if you like.

METHOD

Flake the tuna out of the can into a bowl, then add the zucchini, flour and egg. Mix together to make a batter. If need be, add a dribble of water to loosen the consistency until it resembles heavy cream.

Melt a little of the oil in a frying pan over medium heat. Spoon in large mounds of the batter, leaving some space between each one, as the batter will spread and work itself into a little puddle. Aim for fritters about 3 inches in diameter if you want to make about a dozen—but feel free to just make four big ones instead.

Cook the fritters for 2–3 minutes on each side before lifting them out of the pan and draining on paper towels.

Serve the fritters with a small bowl of soy sauce for dipping.

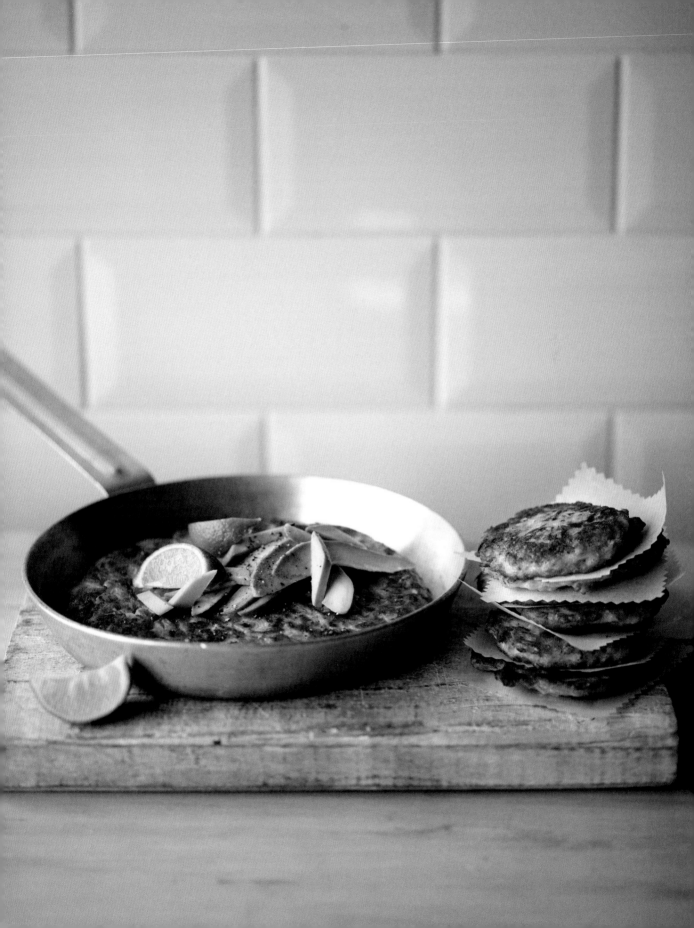

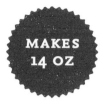

MAKES
14 OZ

INGREDIENTS

14 oz cashews
2 tsp olive or peanut oil
2 tsp ground cumin
1½ tsp smoked paprika

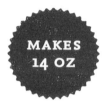

MAKES
14 OZ

INGREDIENTS

14 oz unsalted peanuts
4 tsp wasabi powder
2 tsp olive oil

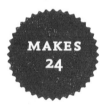

MAKES
24

INGREDIENTS

3 mini tortilla wraps
a few pumps of olive oil spray
2 tsp ground cumin
1 tsp smoked paprika
1 tsp celery salt

SPICED CASHEWS

METHOD

Preheat the oven to 375°F.

Mix all the ingredients together, then tip onto a baking sheet and roast in the oven for 12–15 minutes until the nuts are crisp and lightly colored. Remove from the oven and sprinkle with salt. These spiced nuts will keep in an airtight container for up to 5 days.

WASABI PEANUTS

METHOD

Preheat the oven to 375°F.

Mix all the ingredients together, then tip onto a baking sheet and roast in the oven for 12–15 minutes until the nuts are crisp and lightly colored. Remove from the oven and sprinkle with salt. The wasabi nuts will keep in an airtight container for up to 4 days.

SPICED TORTILLA CHIPS

METHOD

Preheat the oven to 340°F.

Take each tortilla in turn and give it a pump of oil on both sides. Cut the tortilla into quarters, then cut each quarter in half to give you 8 triangles. Lay as many of the 24 triangles onto a baking sheet as you can fit (you might have to use a couple of sheets, or cook the tortilla chips in two batches).

Mix together the spices and salt until they are all well blended, then sprinkle evenly over the triangles. Bake in the oven for 6–7 minutes until lightly golden and crisp.

★ TOP TIP

Nuts are great for a party—and much healthier for you than something like potato chips! But they're still a treat, so don't get too carried away. I recommend a portion of about 1 ounce, no more than once a day.

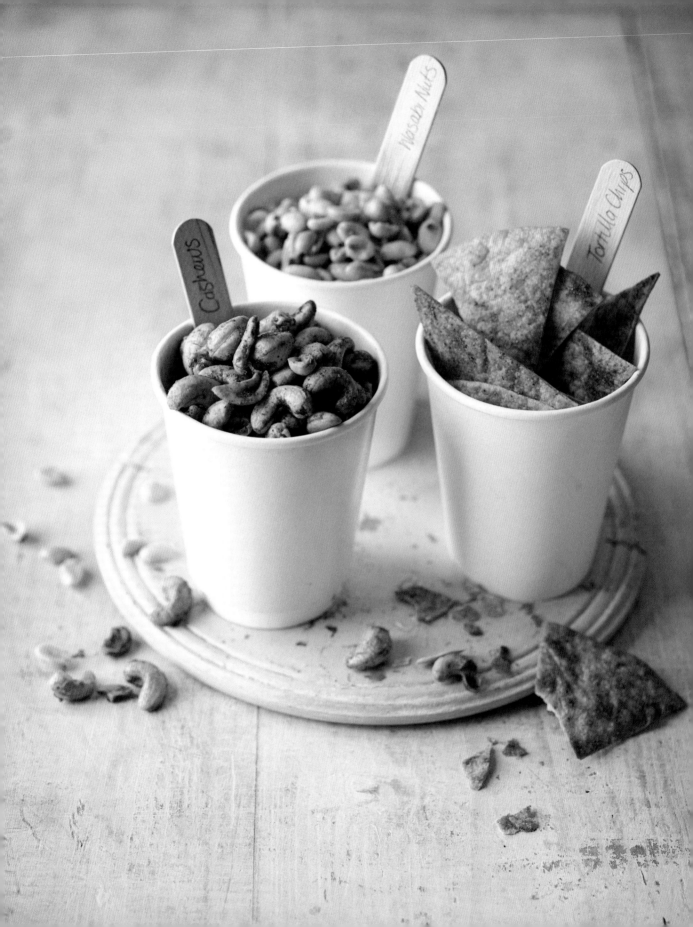

MAKE AHEAD
INGREDIENTS

2 heads of broccoli, broken
  into florets
¼ cup pine nuts
3 tbsp finely grated parmesan
2 bunches of basil, leaves only
1 clove garlic, roughly
  chopped
juice and finely grated zest
  of 1 lemon
5 tbsp olive oil
salt and pepper
chopped raw vegetables,
  to serve

INGREDIENTS

6 oz cream cheese
2 tbsp chopped chives
2 tbsp chopped tarragon
2 tbsp chopped basil
1 small clove garlic, finely
  sliced
6 sun-dried tomatoes, roughly
  chopped
½ cup walnuts, roughly
  crumbled
celery, carrot and cucumber
  sticks, to serve

MIDGET TREE AND PINE NUT PESTO

This is a great snack that will keep in an airtight container in the fridge for up to 3 days. Other green veg, such as kale and spinach, work well too. I like to eat this with chopped cauliflower, carrot and cucumber for dipping.

METHOD

Bring a saucepan of water to a boil. Drop in the broccoli florets and cook for 1 minute. Drain in a sieve or colander, then rinse under cold running water.

Tip the broccoli into a blender and add the pine nuts, parmesan, basil, garlic, lemon juice and zest and olive oil. Season generously with salt and pepper, then pulse until virtually smooth—you will most likely have to do quite a bit of pulsing and scraping.

Serve the pesto with chopped raw vegetables.

WHIPPED-UP HERBY CREAM CHEESE

This is the perfect cheese-lover's snack, and the fresh herbs used in combination are a real winner. This can be made by hand if you don't have a food processor—it just takes a bit more time.

METHOD

Place all the ingredients except the walnuts and the vegetable sticks in a food processor, along with about 2 tablespoons of warm water. Process until totally smooth.

Tip the dip into a bowl, top with the walnuts and then dig in with the celery, carrot and cucumber "spades."

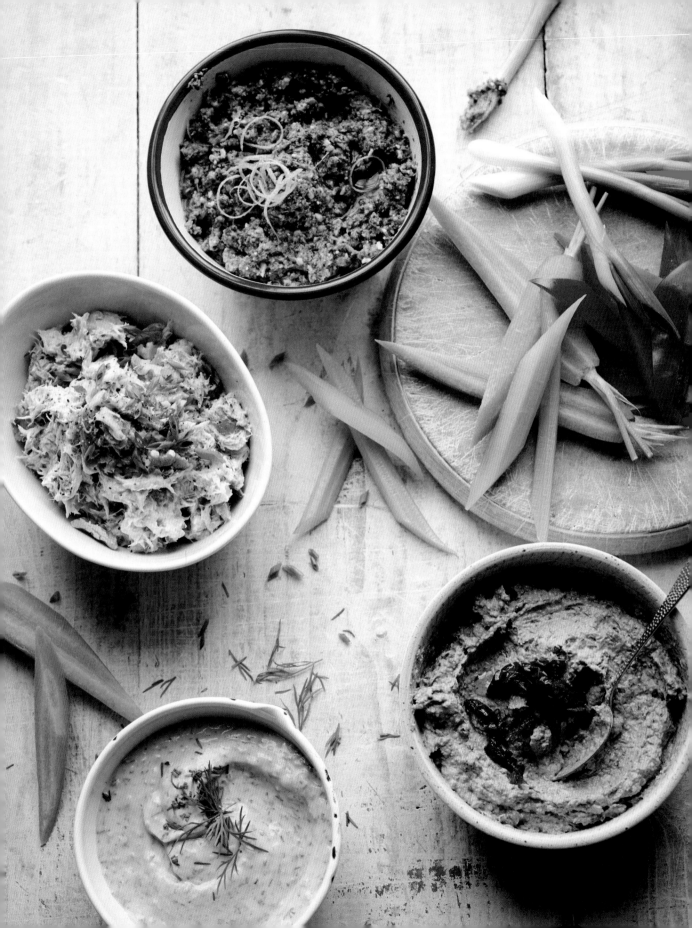

SMOKED MACKEREL PÂTÉ

SERVES 4

Raw cauliflower florets taste amazing with this pâté, which can be kept in an airtight container in the fridge for up to 4 days.

INGREDIENTS

10 oz smoked mackerel
¼ cup crème fraîche
juice of 1 lemon
freshly ground black pepper
small bunch of chives, finely
  sliced
6 tbsp walnuts, roughly
  chopped
chopped carrots, cauliflower
  florets and sliced red bell
  pepper, to serve

METHOD

Remove the skin from the mackerel and, using your fingers, flake the fish into small pieces. Add the crème fraîche and lemon juice, along with a good grinding of black pepper. Use a fork to mix and mash until you're happy with the consistency of your pâté—I like it with a bit of texture.

Stir in the chives, then top the pâté with the walnuts. Serve with the carrots, cauliflower and bell pepper.

AVOCADO RANCH WITH DIPPING STICKS

If you love avocado, this creamy ranch dip will be right up your alley. It only takes about 5 minutes to make and is jam-packed with healthy fats to keep you energized.

INGREDIENTS

1 large avocado, roughly chopped
8 oz full-fat Greek yogurt
juice of 1 lemon
1 clove garlic, grated or finely chopped
small handful of chives, finely chopped
small handful of dill, finely chopped
small handful of parsley, finely chopped
salt and pepper
6 large celery stalks, to serve

METHOD

Place the avocado in a food processor. Add the yogurt, lemon juice, garlic, chives, dill and parsley. Season with salt and pepper, then process until smooth.

Serve the avocado dip with the celery sticks.

★ TOP TIP
SNACK IDEAS

If you don't have time to make a snack, here are a few ideas for you!

★ Scoop of whey protein with water
★ 1 oz nuts
★ 3 oz beef jerky
★ Boiled egg
★ 3 oz fruit (melon, blueberries, strawberries, raspberries, apple or pear). Please limit fruit to one snack per day and try not to have it more than a few times a week because it won't help your fat-burning.

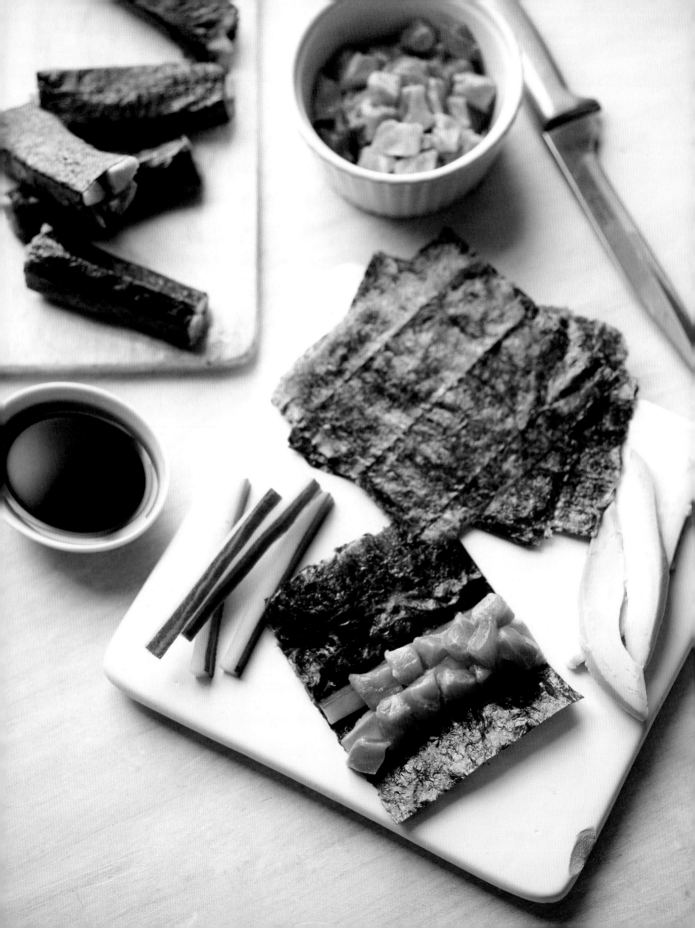

SALMON AND AVOCADO HAND ROLL

Another great snack option that's high in healthy fats. This dish is so impressive you could easily serve it as a starter at a dinner party. Just make sure you get the very freshest fish from your fishmonger—let them know you'll be serving it raw. Anyone with a compromised immune system should avoid raw fish altogether, as should pregnant women.

SERVES 2

INGREDIENTS

- 14 oz raw salmon, cut into ⅓-inch dice—or smaller if possible
- ⅓ inch fresh ginger, finely grated
- 1½ tbsp light soy sauce
- 2 tsp sesame oil
- 2 tsp rice wine vinegar
- 1 avocado, halved and peeled
- 2 large sheets of nori seaweed (about 8 inches square)
- ¼ cucumber, seeded and sliced into 8 sticks

METHOD

Place the salmon, ginger, soy sauce, sesame oil and vinegar in a bowl and mix well.

Cut each avocado half lengthwise into 4 slices, so you have 8 slices of avocado.

Cut each sheet of nori into 4 equal squares.

Spread out your nori squares and lay a slice of avocado in the middle of each one, then sit a cucumber stick alongside. Divide the salmon mixture evenly among the squares of nori, spooning it along the length of the avocado and cucumber.

Dip a finger in some water and dampen the edge of the nori squares so that they will stick.

Roll up your hand rolls and prepare to enjoy a Zen-like taste experience.

BEET PROTEIN BROWNIES

I didn't want to release a cookbook without a few sweet treats. These are yummy, and way healthier than your normal chocolate brownies. But they should still be enjoyed on occasion and not scoffed every day. A slice once a week, after a workout, is fine. These take more like 30 minutes than 15 minutes to make—but hey, you have to earn your treats!

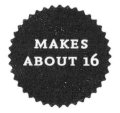

MAKES ABOUT 16

LONGER RECIPE
INGREDIENTS

- 2 cooked and peeled beets (about 5 oz), roughly chopped
- 2 cups minus 2 tbsp ground almonds
- ½ cup chestnut puree
- 5½ tbsp unsweetened cocoa powder
- 2 tbsp honey
- 1 scoop (30g) vanilla protein powder
- 2 tsp vanilla extract
- 4 eggs

METHOD

Preheat the oven to 350°F.

Place all the ingredients in a food processor and process to a smooth batter.

Tip the batter into a lined brownie pan (about 11 × 5 inches) and bake for 18 minutes.

Remove the brownie from the oven and let cool slightly before cutting into squares and chomping down.

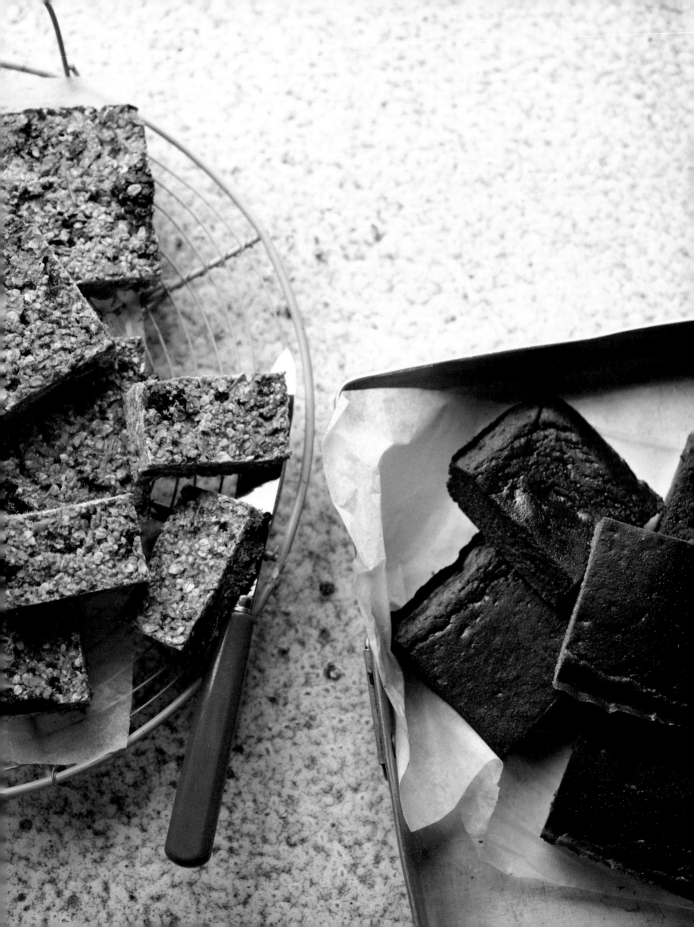

POST-WORKOUT POWER SQUARES

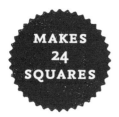

LONGER RECIPE
MAKE AHEAD
INGREDIENTS

12 pitted dates
3½ oz plain rice cakes
2¾ cups rolled oats
1 scoop (30g) vanilla protein
  powder
2 apples, cored and grated
½ tsp baking powder
3½ oz dried cherries, halved

Here's another tasty treat that can be whipped up inside half an hour. But don't forget these aren't for everyday eating. Enjoy them no more than once a week and share them with friends, so you don't scoff all 24 on your own! There's no excuse for "eating them up" so they won't go to waste either, as they'll last for 5 days in an airtight container.

METHOD

Preheat the oven to 325°F.

Bring the kettle to a boil. Cover the dates with boiling water and let soak for 5 minutes.

Pulse the rice cakes in a food processor until they are totally broken down into fine crumbs. Tip them out into a large bowl.

Drain the dates, process in the food processor until smooth and add to the bowl with the rice cakes, along with the remaining ingredients. Mix everything together until thoroughly combined—the mixture can be a bit stiff, so get your hands in there if need be.

Tip the mixture into a lined brownie pan (about 11 x 7 inches) and bake for 25 minutes. Let cool before cutting into squares.

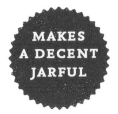

LONGER RECIPE
MAKE AHEAD
INGREDIENTS

**6 oz mixed nuts—I like
cashews, pecans, walnuts,
almonds**
1 tsp ground cinnamon
**1 apple, cored and grated,
skin and all**
2 cups rolled oats
1 tbsp honey
¼ cup raisins

JOE'S GRANOLA

Why buy sugary processed granolas when, with half an hour
to spare, you can make your own healthy version at home?
This goes really well with Greek yogurt and some fresh
berries at breakfast time. Don't rely on it every day, though.
Nothing beats eggs for breakfast.

METHOD

Preheat the oven to 350°F.

Mix all the ingredients except the raisins in a large bowl,
then tip onto a large baking sheet, spreading it out into
a single layer.

Bake for 25 minutes, pulling out the sheet a couple of times
and mixing everything around so the granola toasts evenly.

Remove from the oven and let cool before stirring in
the raisins. The granola will keep in a well-sealed jar for
at least 2 days—although I bet it doesn't last that long!

SERVES 1

JOE'S PROTEIN RICE PUDDING

If you have a sweet tooth, then this is a nice snack to enjoy after a workout, particularly with some fresh berries. Allow about half an hour to make this one.

LONGER RECIPE
INGREDIENTS

½ cup short-grain white rice
2 cups almond milk
1 tbsp honey
1 scoop (30g) vanilla protein
  powder

METHOD

Place the rice, almond milk, honey and ⅔ cup of water in a saucepan. Bring to a boil and simmer for 20–25 minutes, stirring regularly, especially toward the end, when it will become creamy and thick.

Remove from the heat and let cool a little before stirring in the protein powder. Do not add the protein powder with the pan on the heat, or the whey will cook and go lumpy.

Eat the pudding straightaway. Or, for a more indulgent finish, pour into a baking dish and place under a hot broiler until the top is nicely browned and lightly crisp.

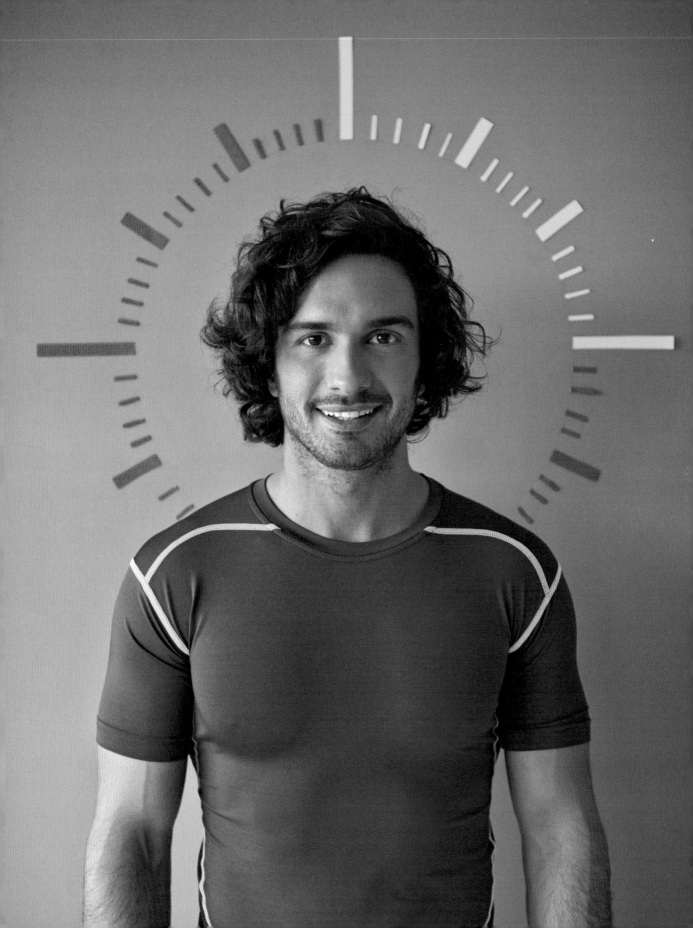

BANANA AND PECAN CUPCAKES

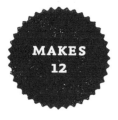

Ready in 20 minutes, these are my favorite treat and quite addictive, so again go easy on them. You won't burn fat eating them every day, so save them for a special treat or make them for a party with friends. The blacker the banana, the better—seriously, totally black is fine for these.

LONGER RECIPE
MAKE AHEAD
INGREDIENTS

3½ oz pecans, plus 12 extra
   for decorating
5 tbsp chestnut puree
3 very ripe bananas, peeled
   and roughly sliced (you need
   about 7 oz flesh)
1½ tbsp honey
1 scoop (30g) vanilla protein
   powder
2 tsp vanilla extract
½ cup ground almonds
4 eggs
¼ cup crème fraîche

METHOD

Preheat the oven to 375°F. Line 12 cups of a muffin tin with paper liners.

Place all the ingredients except the extra pecans and the crème fraîche in a food processor and blend until you have a smooth, runny batter.

Divide the batter evenly among the muffin cups and bake for 18 minutes, or until risen and lightly golden on top.

Let cool, then decorate each cupcake with 1 teaspoon of crème fraîche and a pecan.

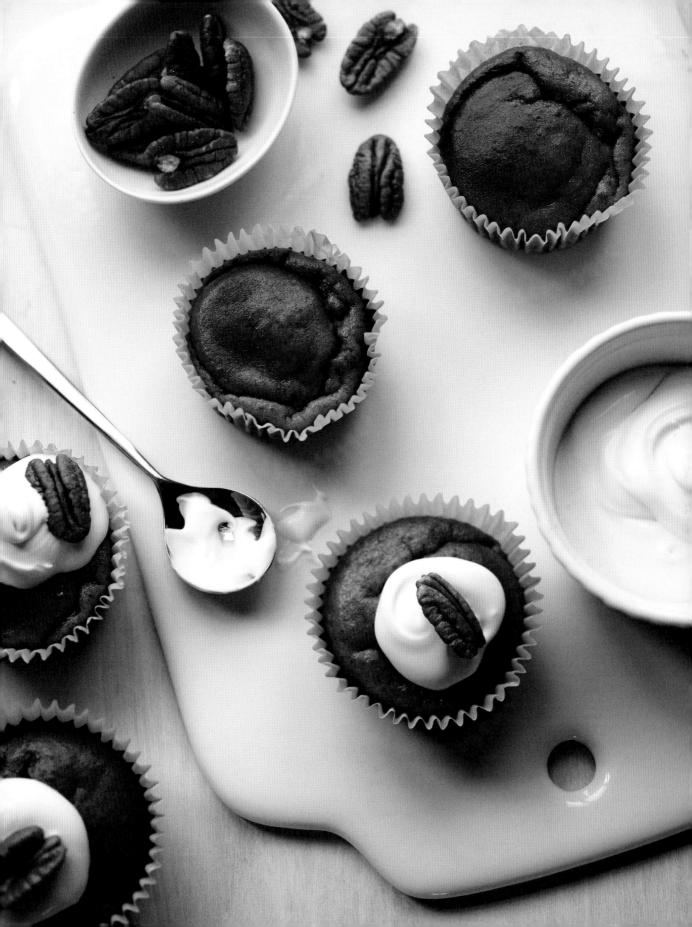

CHEAT'S BANANA AND ALMOND ICE CREAM

LONGER RECIPE
**(quick to make, but needs
4 hours in the freezer)**
MAKE AHEAD

INGREDIENTS

**4 bananas, peeled and cut
into roughly similar-sized
chunks
1 tbsp almond butter
scant ¼ cup almond milk
1 scoop (30g) vanilla protein
powder
toasted sliced almonds, to
serve—optional**

I love ice cream, so I thought I would share this healthier cheat's ice cream recipe with you. Feel free to add other frozen fruit, such as strawberries or raspberries, to mix up the flavor.

METHOD

Line a baking sheet with wax paper and spread the banana chunks over it in a single layer. Place the sheet in your freezer and freeze for a minimum of 4 hours, or until the banana chunks are frozen solid.

Tip the frozen banana into a food processor, along with the almond butter, almond milk and the protein powder, then pulse until virtually smooth.

Serve your cheat's ice cream topped with the toasted almonds, if using.

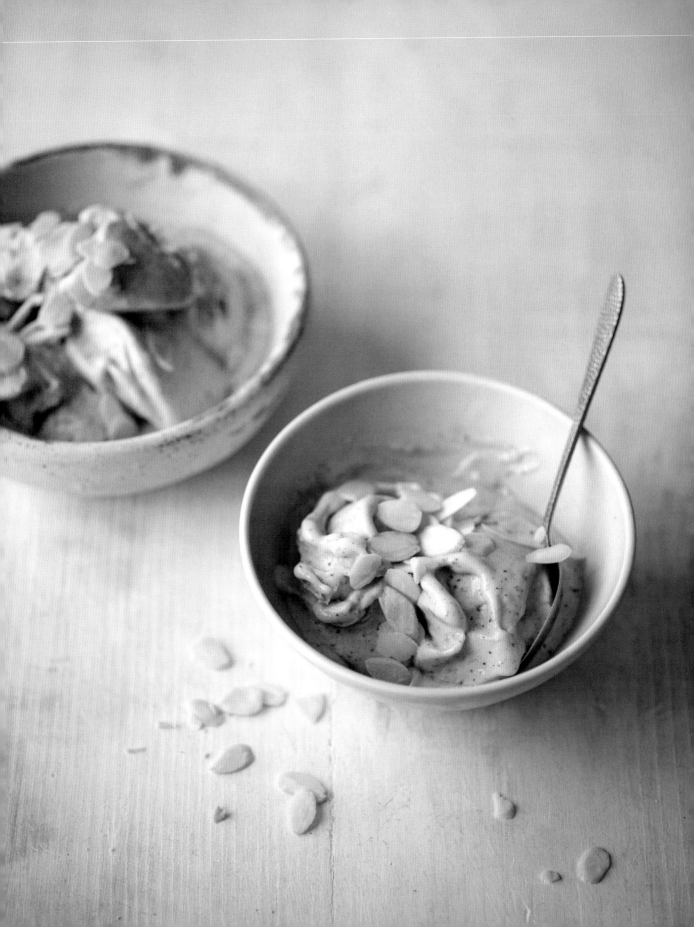

CHOCOLATE AND ALMOND PROTEIN CAKE

SERVES 6

LONGER RECIPE
MAKE AHEAD
INGREDIENTS

4 oz pitted dates
½ cup chestnut puree
2 tbsp unsweetened cocoa
  powder, plus a little extra
  for dusting
1 cup ground almonds
3½ oz chocolate (85% cacao),
  melted
2 scoops (60g) vanilla protein
  powder
4 eggs
finely grated zest and juice
  of 1 orange

Well, I can't pretend this is particularly healthy, but everyone needs a treat sometimes—and, as treats go, this one is packed with nutritional goodness! The higher the percentage of cacao in chocolate, the better it is for you—I've gone for 85% here. And if you don't have chestnut puree, feel free to substitute almond butter. You'll need to allow 30 minutes to make this cake.

METHOD

Preheat the oven to 350°F. Line 9-inch round cake pan with parchment paper.

Bring the kettle to a boil. Pour ⅔ cup boiling water over the dates and let soak for 5 minutes.

Tip the soaked dates, along with their soaking water, into a food processor and puree until smooth. Then add the remaining ingredients and puree into a smooth batter.

Pour the batter into the prepared pan and bake for 20 minutes. The cake will rise in the oven, but collapse again as it cools.

Remove the cake from the pan, dust with the extra cocoa powder . . . and head to the gym for a workout, so you can properly enjoy your treat afterward!

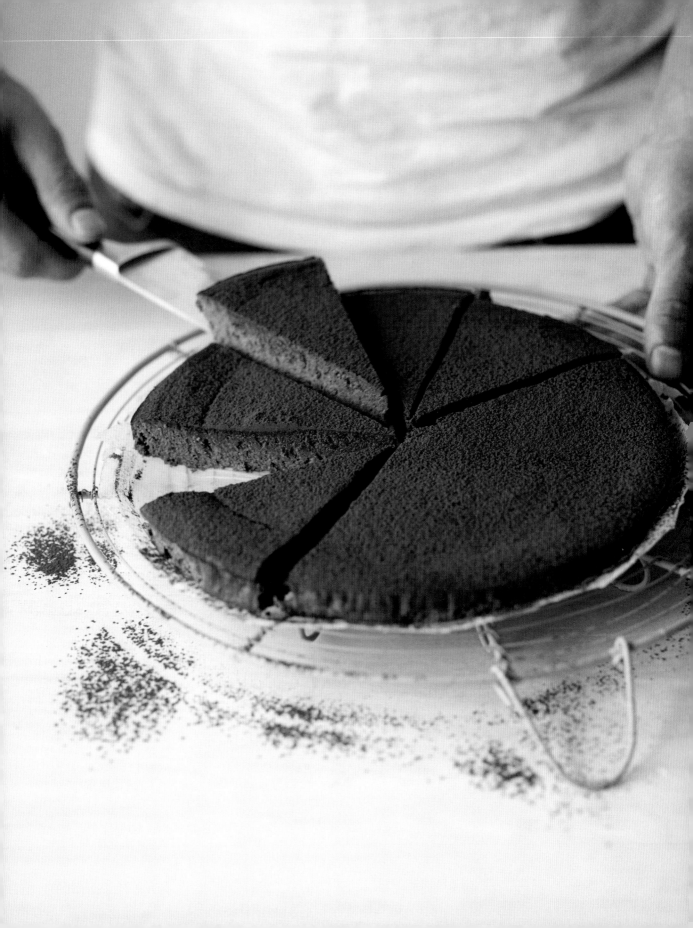

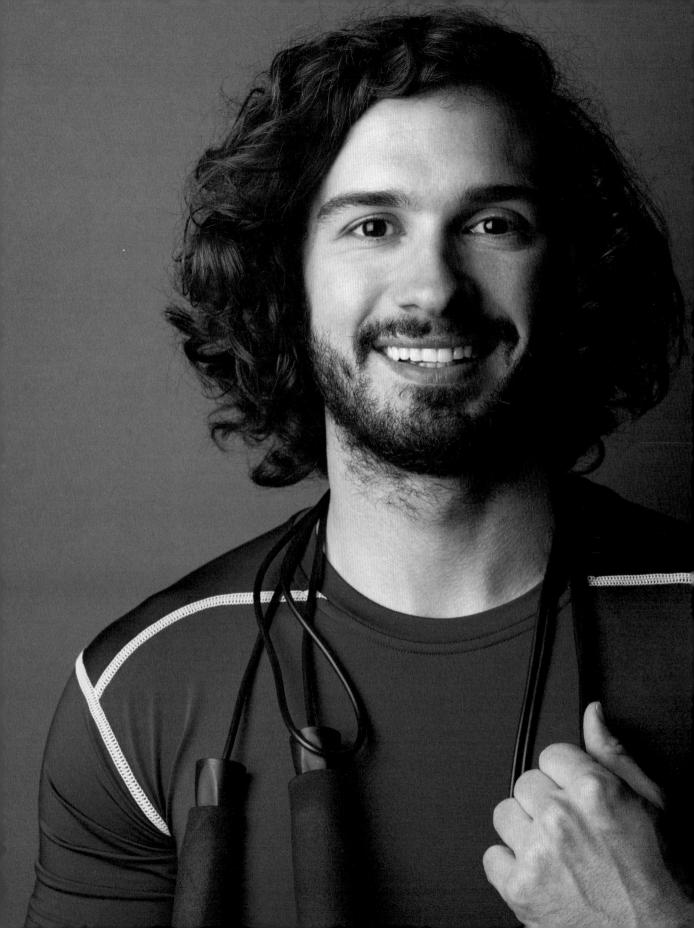

6

BURN FAT AND BUILD LEAN MUSCLE WITH HIIT

HIGH INTENSITY INTERVAL TRAINING (HIIT)

HIIT is one of the most effective training methods for burning fat. It might sound a bit scary, but it's not, as it's all relative to your own fitness and abilities. Everyone on my 90 Day Shift, Shape and Sustain plan, regardless of age or fitness levels, does it—with incredible results. Not only does it burn fat fast, but it also gets you outrageously fit by massively improving your cardio-vascular fitness. Every session should be hard work, but the good news is it's all over in less than 20 minutes and you will feel like an absolute winner after each session. And when your body fat melts away, it's all worth it.

WHAT IS IT?

HIIT involves short bursts of maximal effort, followed by recovery periods of low-intensity activity or rest, i.e., 20 seconds of work, followed by 40 seconds of rest. You repeat this for 15–20 minutes and that's it. Job done. Bye-bye, body fat!

As I said, it's all relative to your fitness levels, so let's take a treadmill, for example: if you're a beginner, HIIT could mean an incline power walk or a jog; if you're much fitter, then it could mean a sprint. The aim is to elevate your heart rate to near maximum during the intense working sets, before letting it recover in the rest periods.

Unlike low-intensity cardio, such as steady jogging, which only burns calories during the actual workout, HIIT burns calories for up to 18 hours afterward. This is known as the after-burn effect, where your body is working hard to repay the oxygen debt in your system and restore itself to a resting state. During this time your metabolic rate is elevated, so your body burns more calories and therefore more fat. The more intense your workout, the greater your oxygen debt will be, so you should always aim to push yourself as hard as possible. Check with your doctor first if you have any health issues. If you can talk, text or tweet during a HIIT session, then you aren't working hard enough—so get in the zone, focus and train like a superhero!

HOW DO I DO IT?

HIIT principles can be applied to any cardio machine, such as a treadmill, cross-trainer, rowing machine or exercise bike, or to

> " Get in the zone, focus and train like a superhero! "

body-weight exercises like burpees, mountain climbers, skipping or sprints.

Choose an exercise or combination of exercises that are suitable for you and that challenge you. You could do the same type of HIIT each time or you can change it up, i.e., rowing machine one day and then cross-trainer the next. As long as you are working hard and enjoying your training, it's all good.

WARM UP

Always carry out an exercise-specific warm-up before starting your HIIT. For example, if you are going to do treadmill sprints, I recommend a power walk or slow jog before you start to sprint. The aim of a warm-up is to prime your muscles and joints for the exercise they're about to perform. This is really important to prevent injuries and ensure you get the most out of your workouts, so don't be naughty and skip your warm-up!

WORKOUT

Once you've warmed up, you can start your HIIT. I find the most effective protocol is a work:rest ratio of 1:2, meaning you rest for twice as long as you work. This allows you to really smash your working set and get a good recovery.

FOR EXAMPLE

> Working set of 20 seconds
> with a resting set of 40 seconds

OR

> Working set of 30 seconds
> with a resting set of 45 or 60 seconds

The effort must come in the working sets, so choose the timings that best suit you. During the resting sets, you can either slow down or come to a complete stop. You will repeat this for 15–20 minutes. It may not seem like much—but trust me, this is enough to create a calorie deficit. And if you fuel your body with the right macronutrients, you will start to see your body transform. Remember that overtraining is NOT necessary, so don't get all carried away by doing two HIIT sessions per day. This will actually be counterproductive for your fat loss. Do one session, do it properly, and you won't want to do it again!

> " DO ONE SESSION, DO IT PROPERLY, AND YOU WON'T WANT TO DO IT AGAIN! "

Here are two workouts for you to try out at home. My advice would be to do both workouts twice each week (so four in total), then add in an extra HIIT, if you fancy it.

WORKOUT 1: *CARDIO HIIT*

This workout involves three body-weight exercises that are guaranteed to get your heart rate up and your body fat melting. You need no equipment and only a small space, so you could do this in the garden or living room.

1. **High knees**

2. **Mountain climbers**

3. **Burpees**

1. **20 seconds High knees 40 seconds rest**

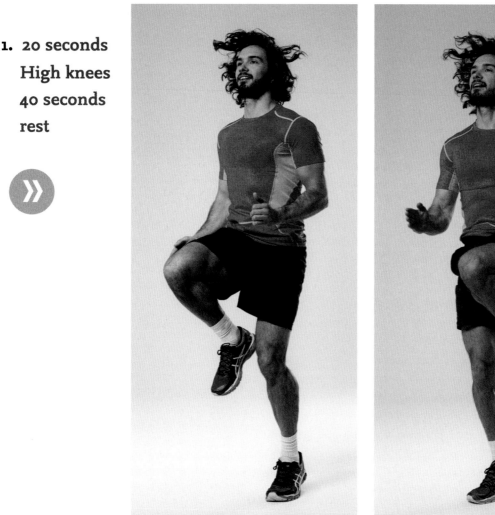

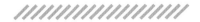

2. **20 seconds Mountain climbers**
40 seconds rest

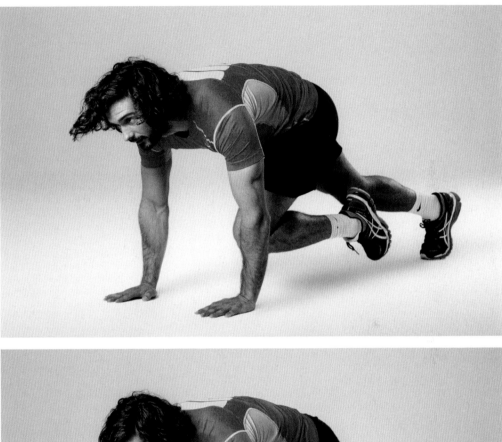

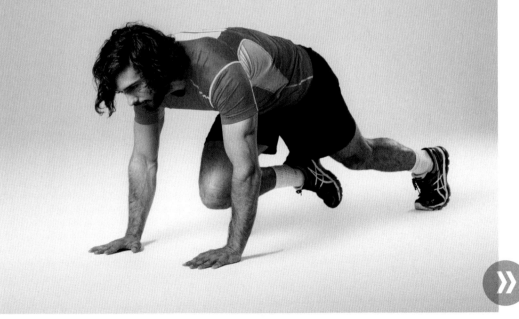

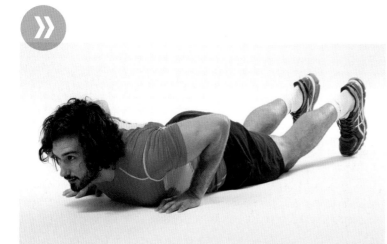

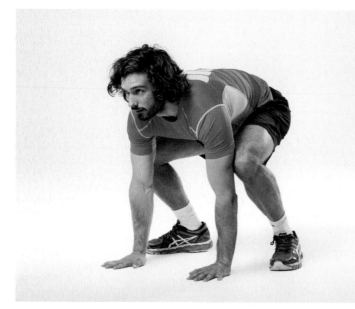

3. 20 seconds Burpees

40 seconds rest

Repeat this circuit 5 times, making a total of 15 minutes. If you find this too easy, work for 30 seconds and rest for 30 seconds.

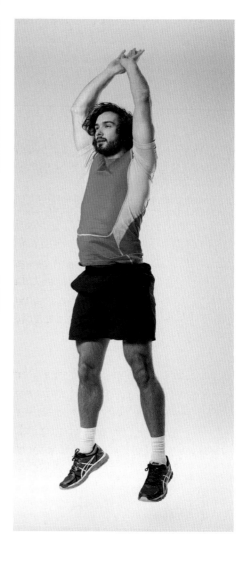

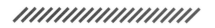

Cool down

Cooling down is really important for your muscles and joints. Have a slow walk or cycle to let your heart rate return to normal. Static stretching or foam rolling can really help reduce your muscle soreness. You may find you experience DOMS (Delayed Onset Muscle Soreness) after your first few sessions. This is totally normal and lasts between 24 and 72 hours. Don't worry, it will pass. It's just your body's way of letting you know you've worked hard, and it will reward you by growing stronger and leaner.

When do I do it?

HIIT cardio is effective at any time of day, so I always recommend doing it when you have the most energy. This could be in the morning before work or late in the evening. Remember, this is your time to "earn" your post-workout carbs.

How often do I do it?

You should aim to do HIIT 4 or 5 days a week for maximum results. If you can't manage that many workouts each week, that's fine—just do what you can and keep a good routine. Remember, though, that on rest days you will be consuming 3 meals from the reduced-carbohydrate menu, so if you want to enjoy your carbs, then you are going to need to find time to smash out a quick HIIT.

Good luck with your workouts. Remember to push yourself and aim to progress each week: this could mean going 0.3m/h faster each week on the treadmill or increasing the weight of your dumbbells by 2 lbs each week. With progression comes strength, and a strong lean body is exactly what you will earn. Be patient and be consistent. Rome wasn't built in a day.

> **" Be patient and be consistent "**

WORKOUT 2: *RESISTANCE HIIT*

/////////////////////////////////

This full-body workout is going to take a bit longer than the HIIT cardio one, as it's going to focus not only on elevating your heart rate, but also on increasing lean muscle with resistance training. By increasing your lean muscle mass, you will increase your metabolic rate, which means you will burn even more fat and can enjoy more food as you get leaner.

All you will need for this is a set of dumbbells for added resistance and an exercise mat. If you are a beginner, start with light weights and aim to increase them as you get stronger. You are going to do the following exercises in a circuit and perform as many reps as possible in 30 seconds. You will then rest for 45 seconds between each exercise. As you get fitter and stronger, you can reduce the rest time to 30 seconds or increase the total number of rounds of 5 full circuits.

1. **Push-ups with dumbbell row**

2. **Dumbbell squats**

3. **Shoulder presses**

4. **Dumbbell lunges**

5. **Bicep curls**

1. 30 seconds Push-ups with dumbbell row

(You can do these on your knees if you prefer.)

45 seconds rest

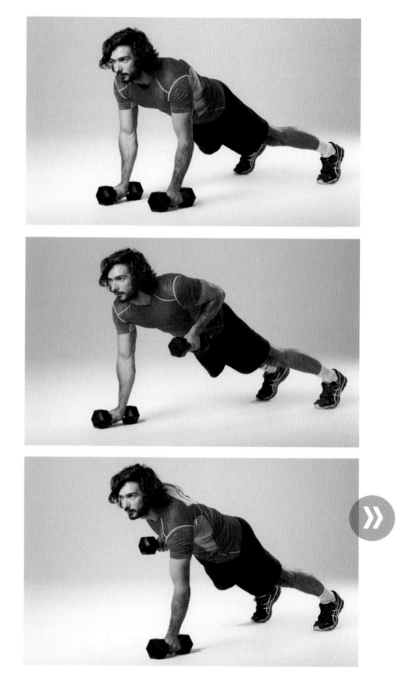

2. 30 seconds
   Dumbbell squats
   45 seconds rest

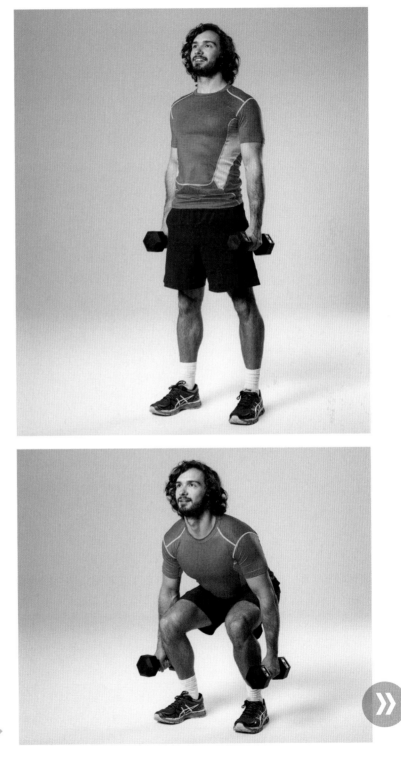

3. 30 seconds Shoulder presses
45 seconds rest

4. 30 seconds Dumbbell lunges
45 seconds rest

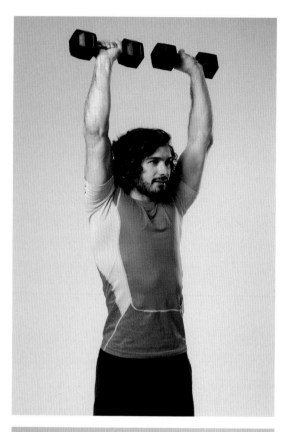

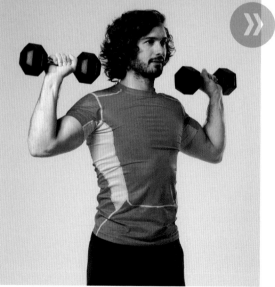

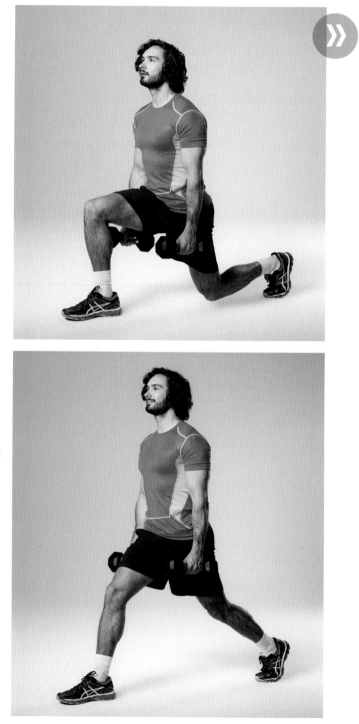

5. **30 seconds**
Bicep curls
45 seconds rest

Repeat this circuit 3–5
times depending on
your fitness level
(approximately 30
minutes).

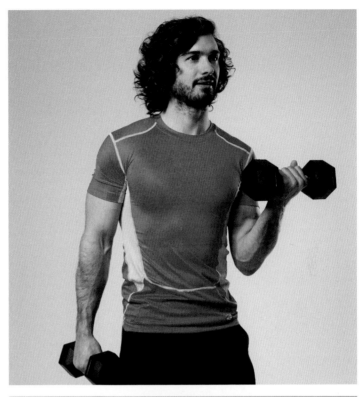

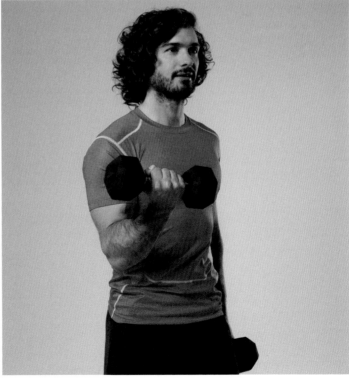

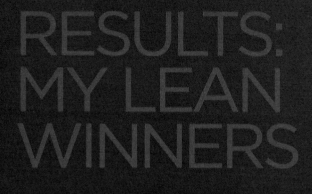

RESULTS: MY LEAN WINNERS

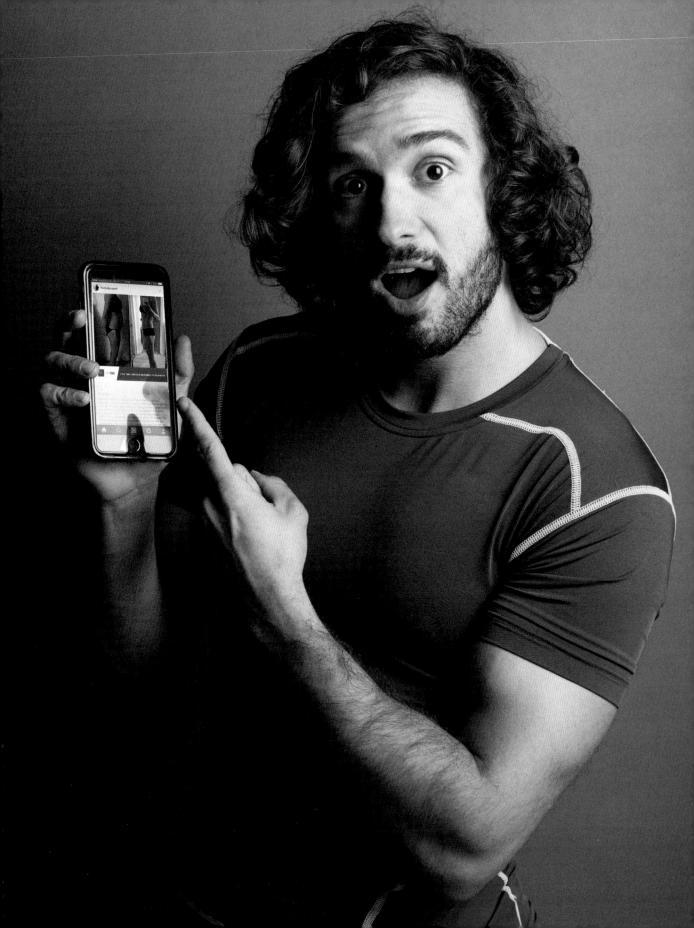

MY LEAN WINNERS

//

For me, one of the most rewarding things about the 90 Day Shift, Shape and Sustain plan is seeing the incredible transformations of my clients, and reading their testimonials. I call them my lean winners—and, although I never actually get to meet them, I'm proud of them all. Not everyone wants to share their stories online and most of those who do want to remain anonymous, but their progress pictures really inspire people. The daily transformations I post on Instagram are one of the reasons so many people have signed up to the plan.

There's nothing better than seeing people of all ages, shapes and sizes succeed in their goals. Often many of them have battled with their weight for years on diets, but in 90 days they transform their body and their relationship with food forever. Knowing that I have educated someone and improved their health and self-confidence is what inspires me to work even harder to help more people. My plan isn't all about weight loss. I have helped people with IBS (irritable bowel syndrome), diabetes, underactive thyroid glands, PCOS (polycystic ovary syndrome) and many other conditions to improve their way of life.

I could fill a whole book with transformations and my graduate heroes, but unfortunately I can only include a handful here. To see more lean winners, visit thebodycoach.co.uk and check out the Transformations gallery, where you'll find thousands of inspirational people, all winning their own little battles and getting fitter and stronger.

Here are just a few of the transformations from the plan (for privacy reasons, I have not included faces or @names), showing some 4-week, 8-week and 12-week transformations, to give you a better idea of the results achieved.

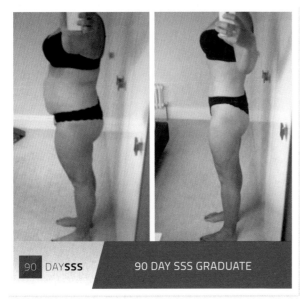

90 DAY**SSS**   90 DAY SSS GRADUATE

★

"The 90 Day SSS plan has changed my life. The education I have received has been invaluable, and I can't recommend this plan enough! I finally feel in control of my diet and my training. I LOVE the gym, and I love the feeling of being full and satisfied from nutritious healthy food. I feel immensely proud, and will be celebrating with a treat tonight before getting right back on that wagon and back in the gym in the morning!!! This is me now: fit, healthy and happy." **Sarah**

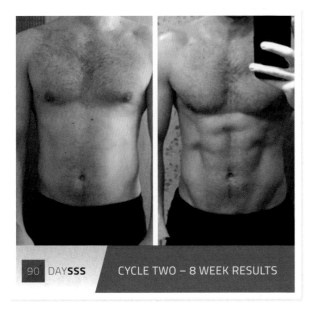

90 DAY**SSS**   CYCLE TWO – 8 WEEK RESULTS

★

"The amount of food was unbelievable. It took a while to get used to it, but once I got the hang of it, it was so simple. My body shape is still changing for the better, and I'm so happy with it. I am so much stronger and feel great!" **Jason**

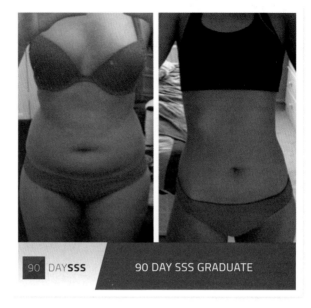

90 DAY**SSS**   90 DAY SSS GRADUATE

★

"I cannot believe the #90daysssplan is already over—it's absolutely flown by. To say I'm extremely pleased with the progress is an understatement! Towards the end of last year I hit a real low. I hated my body and the way I looked, and finally decided to pluck up the courage and do something about it. Life did throw me a few curve balls during cycle 3, so I haven't been able to follow the plan 100%, but I always tried to make up for it the following day with an extra-hard HIIT session. I've done all my workouts from home, so there really are no excuses! Thank you for giving me the confidence I never had." **Kerry**

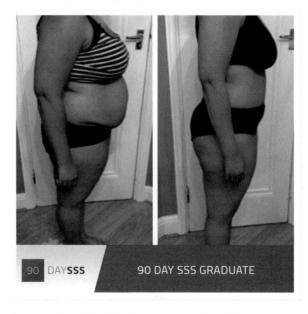

90 DAY**SSS**   90 DAY SSS GRADUATE

★

"I'm so happy that I decided to contact Joe. He has honestly changed my life. I really had zero confidence after having children, but since being on the plan not only has my confidence increased tenfold, it has pushed me to do things in my life that I would have previously been scared to do. Because I'm feeling better, the relationships around me are more positive, and I can play with my children without getting tired. I feel motivated to carry on. The help from Joe has been invaluable and also the kind words from others doing the plan on social media. What he's telling others about healthy fats and body image is so incredibly important, regardless of whether you want to lose weight, gain weight or just get healthy—Joe's plan is a way of life, and the energy and passion behind it make you want to listen. I've even put my scales away. Thank you so much, Joe!" **Jihan**

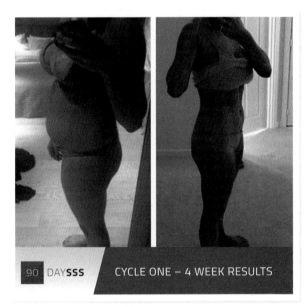

90 DAY**SSS**   CYCLE ONE – 4 WEEK RESULTS

★

"I signed up to the #90dayssplan after seeing the amazing results one of my friends had. I have done every diet you can imagine, but have never seen results like those I got with The Body Coach. I really, really love food and love big portions, so every diet I have ever tried, I have struggled with hunger and cravings, but not on this one. I couldn't quite get my head around how I could eat this much and still lose weight, as I have always thought the less you eat the more you lose. The workouts are tough, but they are only about 25 minutes long, so easy enough to get through. In cycle one I tended to do them at home, following YouTube videos or using an interval timer app—which literally meant that after 25 minutes I was all done and could enjoy my yummy meal." **Sophie**

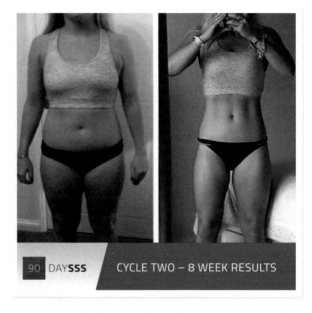

90 DAY**SSS** CYCLE TWO – 8 WEEK RESULTS

★

"The workouts are brilliant—I loved mixing HIIT and using weights, and I could feel myself getting stronger each week. Although I haven't stuck to the food side of things as well as I could have, due to being on Easter holidays, having a few boozy nights out and going away for 5 days, I can honestly say I haven't missed a workout!" **Sarah**

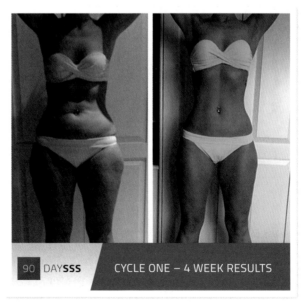

90 DAY**SSS** CYCLE ONE – 4 WEEK RESULTS

★

"I started following Joe on Instagram and signed up straightaway when I saw all the amazing transformation photos. For years I have tried every single low calorie diet and have always been unhappy with my body, especially my tree trunk legs, and was obsessed with the sad step! After seeing my own transformation photo I was shocked that the 'tree trunks' had finally started to shrink. I never thought they would as I always assumed I was just a big-legged girl and no matter what exercise I did or what low-calorie diet I was on, my legs would just stay the same! Considering I used to be obsessed with weighing myself daily, after seeing my photo I think it's amazing that I actually weigh exactly the same as when I started but have lost a whole 10 inches from my body. I definitely will never be obsessed again with what the sad step has to say! I did have a few cheat days, but I stuck to the HIIT sessions 100% which I really enjoyed and can't wait to introduce the weights in cycle 2!" **Rhonda**

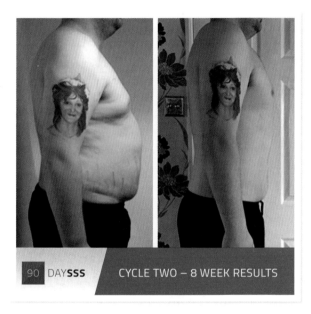

90 DAY**SSS** CYCLE TWO – 8 WEEK RESULTS

★

"For months, even years, I never gave a thought to the food I would eat—and this, combined with no exercise at all and obviously getting older, took a massive toll on my body. Around Christmas last year I looked in the mirror and just realized I really needed to do something. I found Joe purely through chance, with a friend liking one of his videos. I then investigated further and liked the way Joe incorporated humor into fitness and nutrition. This, coupled with the results, made me take the plunge and sign up to the #90daysssplan. Having a complete lack of fitness, I found the first weeks of HIIT tough—I knew I would—but my own determination to plough on, and the support from The Body Coach team, pushed me through. Soon after, I was finding I was enjoying sweating like an absolute beast at 6am . . . strange, I know! Incorporating the weights into cycle two for me was totally alien, having never used weights before! Preparation is most definitely key. I spend around 2 hours in the kitchen on a Sunday, and this sets me up for the week." **Danny**

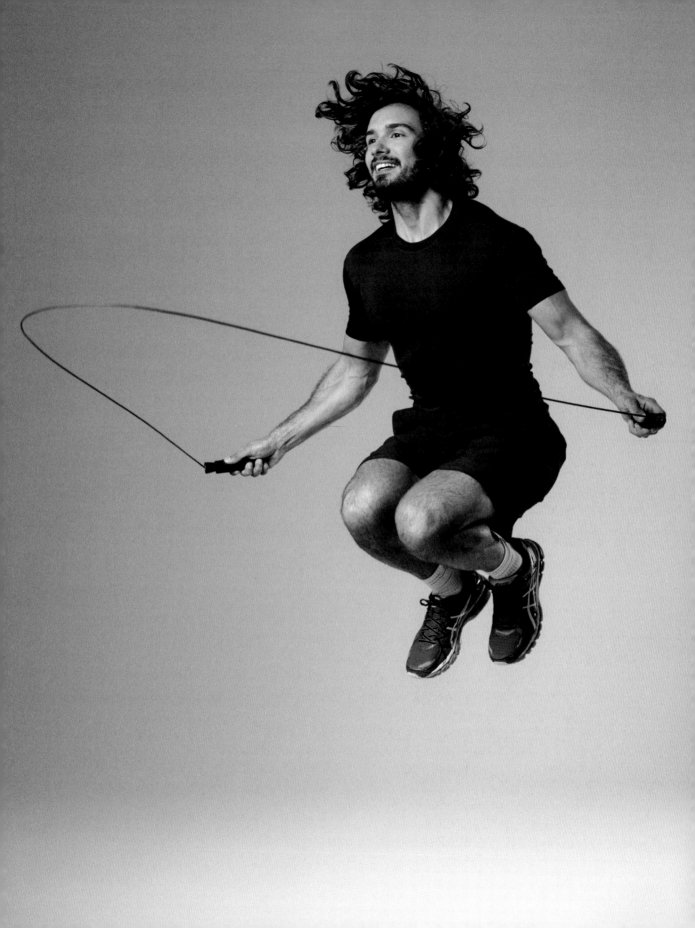

MY TYPICAL WEEK

///

I thought it would be useful to show you how I eat in a typical week, to give you ideas for your own meal planning. You'll notice I eat some of the same meals more than once a week, as I like to batch-cook and keep meals in the fridge for when I'm busy. This really helps me stay on track, as I'm far less likely to grab junk food on the go when I know I have my meals waiting at home when I get in.

You'll also notice that I always have a protein shake with honey immediately after I train. The glucose elevates my blood sugar levels post-workout, triggering the release of insulin, which will send protein to my muscles and start repairing them. When I have a protein shake as a snack at any other time of the day, I don't add honey, but just mix a scoop of protein with some ice and water.

I usually eat my post-workout meal about an hour after I finish a workout, but you can eat sooner or later if you prefer. No matter how early or late you train, you must always choose a carbohydrate-refuel meal after your workout. This is the time your muscles really need to be topped up with glycogen and fed protein to build and repair muscle tissue.

You may think I'm a bit odd eating burgers or stir-fries for breakfast, but I'm giving my body exactly what it needs to burn fat and build lean muscle. Once you start to think outside the cereal box and get over the idea of eating what feels like dinner at breakfast, you'll soon get used to it. Your work colleagues may think you're mad pulling out a chicken stir-fry at 9 A.M., but while they're eating their sugary cereal and gaining body fat, you'll be winning and burning body fat.

The most important thing is to make your meal plan suit your lifestyle, so be flexible in your approach. As long as you consume your 3 meals and 2 snacks at some point during the day, you will burn fat and build lean muscle.

JOE'S PROTEIN SHAKE

1 scoop (30g) vanilla protein
  powder
2¼ tsp honey
3½ oz baby spinach leaves
handful of ice cubes

METHOD

Throw everything in the blender with a good splash of water and blend until smooth.

//////////////////////

	MONDAY	TUESDAY	WEDNESDAY	THURSDAY	FRIDAY	SATURDAY	SUNDAY
Training: am	7am Cardio HIIT		7am Resistance HIIT		7am Resistance HIIT	Rest day	Rest day
Post workout	Joe's protein shake		Joe's protein shake		Joe's protein shake		
Meal 1	Build-up bagel	Poached salmon with bacon	Protein pancakes	Griddled midget trees and spears with eggs	Bad-boy burrito	Griddled midget trees and spears with eggs	Cinnamon reduced-carb oatmeal
Snack	1 oz nuts	Apple	Avocado ranch dip	⅓ cup blueberries	Whipped-up herby cream cheese with celery	1 oz nuts	Protein shake
Meal 2	Lamb koftas with Greek salad	Turkey meatballs with feta	Goan fish curry	Asian duck salad	Ground turkey lettuce boats	Joe's chicken pie	Thai green chicken curry
Snack	Protein shake	Tuna and zucchini fritters	1 oz nuts	Protein shake	1 oz nuts	Whipped-up herby cream cheese with celery	Protein cupcakes
Training pm		6pm Cardio HIIT		6pm Cardio HIIT		Rest day	Rest day
Post workout		Joe's protein shake		Joe's protein shake			
Meal 3	Teriyaki salmon with zucchini noodles	Thai beef stir-fry	Sea bass with spiced cauliflower, peas and paneer	In-a-hurry curry fried rice	Joe's chicken pie	Eat out*	Lamb koftas with Greek salad

*Keeping it lean when eating out

. . . .

One of my favorite things in the world is eating out with family and friends. I have a very simple philosophy when it comes to "cheat" meals. If I know I am going to go for a blow-out meal, then I like to earn it beforehand with a quick 20-minute HIIT session, so I can enjoy the extra carbs and treats as my refuel

meal. If I go out for a meal when I haven't trained, then I try to stick to just fats and proteins and leave the carbs alone, opting for something like grilled steak or fish with lots of vegetables and a big drizzle of olive oil. These small food choices really will make a big difference over time and allow you to stay lean.

	MONDAY	TUESDAY	WEDNESDAY	THURSDAY	FRIDAY	SATURDAY	SUNDAY
Training: am							
Post workout							
Meal 1							
Snack							
Meal 2							
Snack							
Training pm							
Post workout							
Meal 3							

USE THIS TABLE TO PLAN YOUR OWN MEALS AND WORKOUTS FOR THE WEEK

Prepping like a boss

. . . .

I hope you love the food in this book as much as I do, and get inspired to start cooking more and prepping like a boss so you can achieve the healthy body you want. Just remember that fat loss takes time, dedication and consistency. You can and will get lean—just keep working hard and make it a habit to eat the Lean in 15 way.

LEAN IN 15 HEROES

//

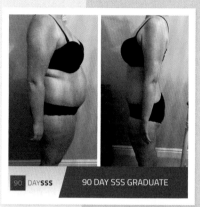
90 DAY SSS GRADUATE

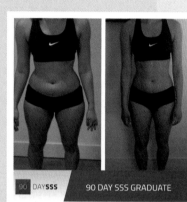
90 DAY SSS GRADUATE

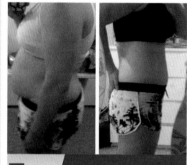
CYCLE ONE—4 WEEK RESULTS

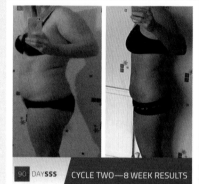
CYCLE TWO—8 WEEK RESULTS

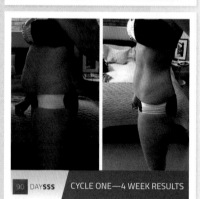
CYCLE ONE—4 WEEK RESULTS

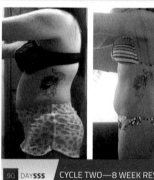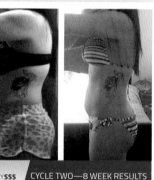
CYCLE TWO—8 WEEK RESULTS

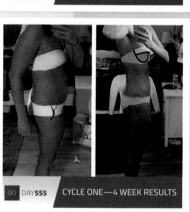
CYCLE ONE—4 WEEK RESULTS

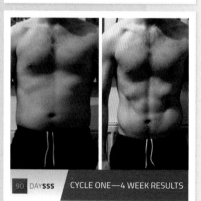
CYCLE ONE—4 WEEK RESULTS

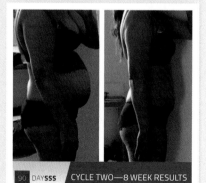
CYCLE TWO—8 WEEK RESULTS

90 DAY SSS GRADUATE

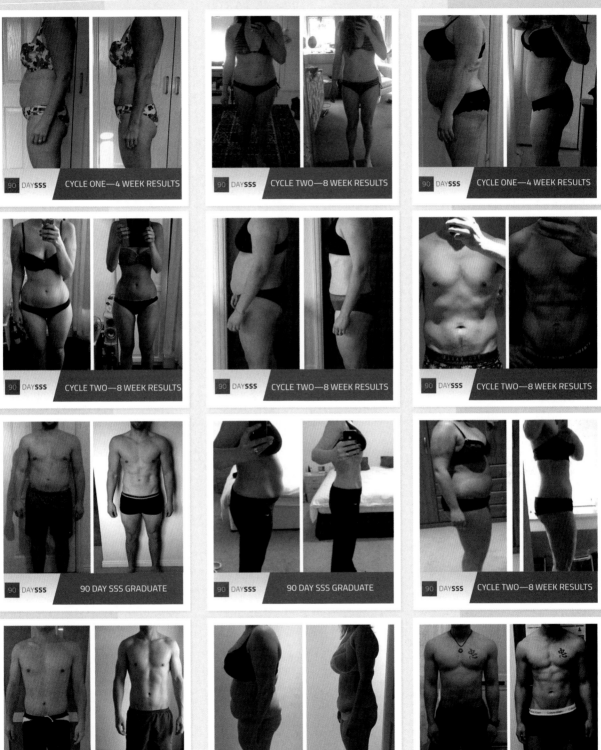

90 DAY**SSS** CYCLE ONE—4 WEEK RESULTS

90 DAY**SSS** CYCLE TWO—8 WEEK RESULTS

90 DAY**SSS** CYCLE ONE—4 WEEK RESULTS

90 DAY**SSS** CYCLE TWO—8 WEEK RESULTS

90 DAY**SSS** CYCLE TWO—8 WEEK RESULTS

90 DAY**SSS** CYCLE TWO—8 WEEK RESULTS

90 DAY**SSS** 90 DAY SSS GRADUATE

90 DAY**SSS** 90 DAY SSS GRADUATE

90 DAY**SSS** CYCLE TWO—8 WEEK RESULTS

90 DAY**SSS** 90 DAY SSS GRADUATE

90 DAY**SSS** CYCLE ONE—4 WEEK RESULTS

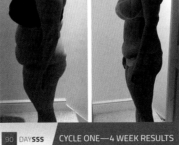

90 DAY**SSS** CYCLE ONE—4 WEEK RESULTS

INDEX

ACKNOWLEDGMENTS

I would like to start by thanking everyone who has ever completed my 90 Day plan and followed me on social media. Because of you, I've been able to build a following, spread my message and have the opportunity to release this book. Without you, I would just have been a dude in a kitchen talking to midget trees, so thanks for sticking around and sharing my videos with others.

I would also like to say thank you to all my friends and family who love and support me in my goals.

See you in June for *Lean in 15*, volume 2—*The Shape Plan*.

CREDITS

Publisher: Carole Tonkinson
Assistant Editor: Olivia Morris
Design: Ami Smithson
Desk Editor: Claire Gatzen
Food Photography: Maja Smend
Fitness Photography: Glen Burrows
Food Styling: Bianca Nice
Prop Styling: Lydia Brun
Makeup Artist: Jo McKenna